'This book is an excellent resource for chronic pain patients. The book educates patients about pain in ways that are simple to understand, and then offers a large number of practical suggestions for individuals with pain. Most pain patients are unaware of the large number of things they can do themselves to better manage their pain and as such become overly reliant on doctors and healthcare systems. But our healthcare systems often make individuals with chronic pain worse rather than better, by offering excessive diagnostic testing, unhelpful surgery or injections, or potentially harmful drugs.'
Daniel Clauw, MD, Professor of Anesthesiology, Medicine, and Psychiatry and the Director of the Chronic Pain and Fatigue Research Center at The University of Michigan

'As a primary care physician responsible for a very large patient panel, I was often overwhelmed when confronted with patients who were struggling with chronic pain. My resources were usually limited to an order for labs or imaging, a referral form, and my trusty prescription pad. Reading Dr. Parks' insights about an alternative way to view chronic pain has been eye-opening and provides a more optimistic approach in understanding and helping empower my patients. With information about the neuroscience of chronic pain and the adaptation of a more mind-body approach, I have realized that much of my previous treatment may not have been as beneficial as intended. This book should be mandatory reading for all medical students.'
Lyn Hulst, MD, Staff Physician, Mary Free Bed Pain Rehabilitation Center

'If you are on the roller coaster of medical treatments without relief, you need to hear what Dr. Parks has to say. If you are fed up and frustrated with pain and don't like the life you are living, you need to hear what Dr. Parks has to say. It will not be easy. You will need to reconsider much of what you believe to be true, but the payoff will be well worth it.'
Mike Terrell, PT, MSPT, Cert. MDT, Certified Therapeutic Pain Specialist

'I highly recommend this book. It's written in plain language that all of us can understand. Read it and you will learn that you can think of pain as a resource, a mislabeled physiological process, or just an event, it's your choice. You will also begin to see that you already have competence in dealing with pain.'
Kevin Polk, Ph.D., Creator of The ACT Matrix

T0271485

'Finally, a book that gives real hope to pain sufferers and their physicians. This book should change the paradigm for pain treatment. Patients who read it should immediately give a copy to their physician or find a physician with a similar perspective. Physicians who read it will have the rationale and tools for pursuing a better treatment path. The book is full of ideas for both patients and healthcare professionals to work together to relieve suffering.'
Charles Dolph, Ph.D., Senior Professor of
Psychology at Cedarville University

'This book provides a clear understanding of the causes of pain and what happens in the brain that produces the sensation of pain. Dr. Parks provides those with chronic pain new hope through understanding and skill-building to take back their lives that have often been derailed by chronic pain and the traditional medical treatments of chronic pain. While the book is aimed at those with chronic pain, it would be hugely beneficial for medical and mental health professionals who provide treatment to the large population who struggle with chronic pain issues.'
Marcia K. Wiinamaki, PsyD, Licensed Clinical Psychologist

'Dr. Parks lays out what is so important for persons with chronic pain to understand as they work toward re-engaging in purposeful activity. With goals of participating once again in activities at home, work, and leisure, building on smaller successes can lead to greater confidence. It is essential to understand how one's own thoughts, both positive and negative, can impact the recovery of function and level of pain. Clinically, when our treatment team sees patients apply the strategies Dr. Parks describes, we see patients improve their functioning and report less pain. The changes that occur are noticed by family members and friends as well.'
Mark DeKraker, MS, OTR/L

'This dynamic book provides key insights to help a chronic pain patient move from despair to discovery. Dr. Parks sets the reader on a path of transformation. Learning the real story behind chronic pain frees you to redirect your energies toward reclaiming your life.'
Lori Caldwell-Ritsema PA-C, Center for
Adolescent and Child Neurology

CHRONIC
PAIN
REHABILITATION

Active Pain Management to Reclaim
the Life you Love

DR. EVAN PARKS

Foreword by Dr. James Hudson

First published in the USA in 2020 by Wandering Words Media

First published in Great Britain in 2024 by Headline Home,
an imprint of Headline Publishing Group

1

Trade paperback ISBN 978 1 0354 2325 5
eISBN 978 1 0354 2327 9

Typeset in 12.75/17.75pt Adobe Caslon Pro by Jouve (UK), Milton Keynes

Printed and bound in Great Britain by Clays Ltd, Elcograf S.p.A.

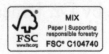

MIX
Paper | Supporting
responsible forestry
FSC® C104740

HEADLINE PUBLISHING GROUP
An Hachette UK Company
Carmelite House
50 Victoria Embankment
London EC4Y 0DZ

www.headline.co.uk
www.hachette.co.uk

For Carrie, my loving companion
on the journey through life

CONTENTS

FOREWORD

Pain is a part of the human experience.

All of us experience acute pain from injuries or illnesses that are just part of life: headaches, sore throats, sprains and strains, bruises and abrasions. More serious pain can come with fractures, accidents, surgeries, cancers, and arthritis. As long as the pain goes away as we heal, we can deal with it. It is when the pain becomes truly chronic that we struggle because that is when the usual treatments offered by modern medicine seem to lose their effectiveness. Patients in chronic pain often end up with multiple surgeries, multiple injections and medications, and sometimes implanted spinal cord stimulators or other high-tech devices often with only temporary benefit.

This book is about another way, a truly biopsychosocial approach, also known as a mind-body approach. It is an important book because our medical education system has not done a good job of teaching our health care teams about the most recent findings in pain science and patients are often left to search for answers themselves. Dr. Parks is here, educating us about how to approach our own pain in a way that reduces the suffering and anguish that chronic pain can produce.

A study by Johns Hopkins University showed that the economic costs of chronic pain exceed the costs of cancer, diabetes, or heart disease and can be as high as $635 billion dollars per year. With each of these other conditions we have well-defined guidelines for treatment, and over the past three decades we have made major advances in treatment. With pain, however, we have widespread disagreement on how it ought to be treated and we have not demonstrated any significant progress in controlling pain. Instead, we have seen a catastrophic rise in prescriptions for opioid pain relievers, opioid overdose deaths, and no reduction in overall reported pain levels or disability during those past three decades.

I have treated chronic pain since 1983, and the most progress we have seen in this field has been related to educating patients about the body's nervous system and how it handles pain—teaching skills for calming the nervous system when pain occurs. These skills have been more effective than pain medications, injections, or passive therapies. There is nothing magical about this approach. It requires dedication to learning the principles and techniques and practicing them. Dr. Parks has laid out approaches to pain that have proven to help individuals gain control of their pain. It doesn't result in a pain free life, but it keeps pain from taking over our lives. We can focus on living again—on the pursuits and activities that are the most important and meaningful to us. If this is what you are looking for, you have come to the right place. I wish you success as you begin to take back your life.

James D. Hudson, MD
Medical Director
Mary Free Bed Hospital Pain Rehabilitation Programs

INTRODUCTION

This book is about understanding how chronic pain develops and ways you can manage pain and get back to living the life you love. Three personal stories of individuals with chronic pain will illustrate how active pain management strategies bring lasting change. Their stories will give you hope in your struggle with pain. You will learn about:

- David, after a serious work-related injury, had several back surgeries that left him in constant pain. Robbed of sleep, he was convinced he would never work again.
- Rachel, a young mother and businesswoman with fibromyalgia, feared her life was over due to chronic fatigue and the pain throughout her body.
- Nancy, who injured her neck in a car accident, had headaches, migraines, and neck and shoulder pain for twenty years. She had given up hope for finding relief.

ISOLATION AND MISUNDERSTANDING

David, Rachel, and Nancy each had problems finding the right medical care to address their specific types of chronic pain. Even though they worked with different doctors and healthcare providers, they all experienced similar frustrations with a medical system that misunderstood the unique challenge of chronic pain.

Though the medical care they received for other health problems came with clear diagnoses, David, Rachel, and Nancy were never given an explanation for their persistent pain. Chronic pain was never explained beyond the basic, "Well, this happens sometimes." Their doctors continued to provide the standard treatments for chronic pain even though the surgeries, injections, medications, implanted devices, and therapies were not working. Medical interventions continued even when there were signs the pain was becoming worse. To add to their disappointment and stress, they were told that the pain might be all in their heads.

This book is not written to blame doctors or the healthcare system. Healthcare professionals are dedicated to relieving suffering and do not want to cause more problems for their patients. But many physicians feel they are doing more harm than good when one treatment after another fails to help their patients manage chronic pain. After several attempts at treating chronic pain with standard, recommended care, many physicians become frustrated and suspect the problem is psychological, shifting blame to the patient.

Chronic pain sufferers also face disappointment with friends, family, and co-workers. David, Rachel, and Nancy have each heard: "Oh, you're still not feeling well? I thought you were better now. You look fine!" People suffering from chronic pain feel isolated due to a general lack of understanding from others. They often lose contact with friends and their ability to work. Some even lose their homes and marriages.

REASONS FOR HOPE

For many people who have suffered from chronic pain for years, being offered hope can be upsetting. Too often, medical care providers suggest treatments that only leave pain sufferers disappointed. Patients are often told that a new medication, a different type of injection, one more surgery, or an implanted stimulator device is the key to relief. But when a pain sufferer has tried them all, hope runs thin.

If you are suffering from chronic pain, there is hope. This hope is not based on new medical interventions, but on a clear scientific understanding of how chronic pain develops. I will help you understand where chronic pain comes from and what you can do to learn to live with the nervous system you have. This hope is based on three principles: (1) understanding how the mind and body operate; (2) developing pain management tools to manage your chronic pain and reduce your pain sensations; and (3) developing emotional flexibility that keeps you moving forward even when pain is in your way.

YOUR GUIDE

I am a clinical psychologist specializing in pain management. The hospital where I work is one of the few that offers a comprehensive, multidisciplinary program for chronic pain. Many of the patients we see already have had extensive pain treatment. For some, their primary care doctor has become frustrated by the lack of change in pain symptoms. So many patients come to us from doctors who have said: "I don't know what to do with you anymore. We have tried everything. You have seen the neurologist and the rheumatologist, been to pain clinics, had chiropractic care, tried all the pain medications, and had surgery." As a result, patients arrive at our pain program feeling that everyone has given up on them and that there is no hope left.

By working in a teaching hospital that is training the next generation of physicians, I see the best treatment practices. The research that guides the future of chronic pain rehabilitation is happening here. We also hear from our patients about a wide range of pain treatments and interventions they have been subjected to over the years. This book condenses all that cutting-edge information and puts it into plain, easy-to-understand language. With knowledge from neuroscience, pain psychology, and rehabilitation, you will learn to get back to living an active, meaningful life.

WHAT YOU WILL LEARN

This book will take you through the three steps of active pain management:

- Step One: Understand acute and chronic pain
- Step Two: Calm the central nervous system
- Step Three: Develop emotional flexibility

You need the pieces of your chronic pain puzzle put together so you can make sense of them. As you make your way through this book, you will gain the knowledge necessary to live well, even with the challenges you face.

I care for people with chronic pain. When I sit down with new patients, I can see years of frustration, pain, and discouragement written on their faces. When Nancy arrived for her appointment, it was easy to see that after twenty years of chronic pain, she was worn out. She had lost much of her ability to engage in a meaningful life. Nancy was hurting both physically and emotionally.

What I enjoy so much about my work is being able to see people like Nancy start living life again and pain patients start doing what is important to them. This dramatic turnaround in a person's life makes the work I do exciting. I am fascinated by the way the brain can change and rewire itself. The information in this book will help you rewrite the story of your life. I have seen so many people change their lives that I wanted to outline these pain transforming principles so others could experience these changes for themselves.

As you read this book, you will gain a better understanding of how chronic pain develops and acquire the tools you need to get your life back again. You will understand the mind-body connection, ways to calm your oversensitive nervous system, and how to manage the stress.

A WORD OF CAUTION

This book is for a specific audience—people who already have a good healthcare team in place. Pain is a symptom that everyone needs to take seriously. Some readers may hope to learn a non-medical approach to pain management rather than see their doctor about their aching back. This book is not for you. Pain can point to serious medical problems, even when the pain is a common headache. Only a physician who knows you well can make sure that the aches and pains you have are worth further investigation.

Furthermore, if you rely on alcohol, opioids, muscle relaxers, anxiety medication, or other legal or illegal drugs, please get medical help and consider reducing your dependence on these and other medications to manage pain. Medications provide a passive form of pain management and may not be enough to manage your pain effectively or move you in the direction of health and well-being.

The approach presented in this book is active—you'll learn how to manage pain yourself. If you have diabetes, obesity, traumatic brain injury, kidney disease, high blood pressure, emphysema, COPD, or other chronic medical conditions, consult with your medical provider before you apply the principles in this book. Talk to your doctor about your diet as well; vitamin and mineral deficiencies can contribute to pain, as does not drinking enough water.

MAKE A COMMITMENT

You have a choice to make as you read this book. One option is to flip through the pages, looking for topics that seem interesting, reading a little, but not acting on what you read. After a few weeks or months, you likely will still have the chronic pain symptoms you do now. Another option is to make a commitment, set aside the time to study this book, and put into practice the ideas outlined here. If you do this, you will develop skills that help you manage pain, calm your nervous system, and become more engaged in life. Your progress might be slow, but you will make progress. As you become less focused on pain, you will see the changes in your life, the same changes I have seen in so many people's lives who were once without hope.

Why put up with one more day, one more week, or one more month of misery? The help you need is here in the neuroscience of how chronic pain operates. With these scientific principles, you can move toward a healthier life and away from the problems that cause pain.

STEP ONE

UNDERSTAND PAIN

The greatest mistake physicians make is that they attempt to cure the body without attempting to cure the mind; yet the mind and body are one and should not be treated separately!

—Plato (428 BCE–348 BCE)

Any man could, if he were so inclined, be the sculptor of his own brain.

—Santiago Ramón y Cajal (1852–1934)

Understanding pain requires learning about the different types of pain, the function that pain serves, and how the experience of pain can drastically change over time.

In this section, we will take our first steps toward effective pain management by learning how pain operates and where it comes from. You will learn why the standard medical approach to chronic pain generally fails and can actually make chronic pain worse. Armed with the latest brain science, you will learn how to help the brain overcome its oversensitivity to pain through a step-by-step process designed to calm the central nervous system.

1

• • •

IT'S NOT YOUR DOCTOR'S FAULT

David arrived at my office angry and out of patience with the medical care system. With each past medical intervention, he was given the same promise: "Don't worry, David. After this, you will be better than new." This reassurance was given when he received surgery, steroid injections, and physical therapy, and when he was implanted with an electric stimulating device in his back. Some of these interventions brought relief, but only for a short period of time.

As the months passed without lasting relief, David's hope began to drain away, and discouragement, frustration, sleep problems, and lack of energy began to set in. David did not even know he was depressed or what was causing the changes in his mood and outlook on life. All he knew for certain was that he felt terrible, both emotionally and physically. For the first time in his life, he did not feel like living anymore, which confused him. He saw himself as a strong person with a supportive family. Why would he feel like giving up?

David's story, like that of so many others, started with the physically demanding work he did every day for years. While working in a warehouse and moving large wooden pallets of building supplies, he pulled on the handle of the powerful hydraulic jack to get the 1,000-pound load moving. That is when he heard it, that awful sound of something popping in his back. He fell to his knees and let out a scream. His workmates ran to find the factory manager, who came to the scene of the accident and called an ambulance. That was David's last day of work and the first day of a long journey of doctor visits, exams, injections, physical therapy, and surgeries.

After two years of being off work, losing workers' compensation, and multiple failed attempts to get disability benefits from the government, David was desperate. At twenty-eight years old, he felt his life was over. He came to the pain center without hope, angry at life, and convinced that this next round of treatment was going to be just like his last several attempts—a complete waste of time.

STANDARD MEDICAL TREATMENT

This account of David's chronic pain probably brings your own stories to mind. We all know people who have been injured and then struggle to find the help they need to deal with their ongoing pain. You might have experienced something like this yourself. If you have, then you have probably asked a very reasonable question, "Why has my medical treatment not helped relieve my pain?"

David spent hours talking with friends and family about his failed treatments. The pain and the worry kept him awake at night and gave him an ulcer during the day. Without going into the specifics of David's medical history, let me suggest what may have gone wrong with his health care: The medical treatments he received focused only on a specific mechanical problem—the condition of his spine—but not on promoting the health of the tissues, muscles, and nerves, or on calming his overly sensitive nervous system. As we will see, standard medical interventions for chronic pain focus mostly on using medical interventions that doctors are familiar with, such as medications, injections, medical devices, and surgeries, rather than moving a person toward healing, health, and well-being by calming the nervous system and reducing pain.

If standard medical interventions do not always help with chronic pain, what is the average person supposed to do? Most injured people are not trained in medicine, physical therapy, or pain science and would have a hard time coming up with alternatives and options for their own medical care. The doctor writes the prescription, and we take our medicine—whether we like it or not. But it is not the doctor's fault that they approach chronic pain in this manner. Doctors are trained to follow standard procedures to address the typical kind of medical problems they are expected to treat. The same goes for treating chronic pain. Physicians have been educated to approach such treatment based on the recommendations of professional medical societies, research, and guidelines from the federal government.

Even though there are standard medical treatments for chronic pain, not everyone follows their doctor's advice to take more medications or have surgery. I have talked with many people who have thought through their medical options and decided that their only alternative was to suffer in pain. These people do not believe that surgery will solve their problems or fear they may become addicted to prescribed opioid pain medications.

Avoiding surgeries, injections, and medications does not necessarily lead people with chronic pain to health and well-being. In fact, that's a good way to make sure chronic pain sticks around. What both patients and healthcare professionals need is a clearer understanding of how pain works. Based on the scientific knowledge of how the brain produces pain and how nerves and tissue recover from injury, we can choose pain management approaches that help address the specific problem of chronic pain, which is its own unique type of mind-body problem.

THINKING ABOUT PAIN DIFFERENTLY

Think about how David's pain was viewed by his previous medical treatment team, which offered the surgeries, medication, and injections. His entire treatment was based on the belief that a specific problem (e.g., a pinched nerve, a slipped disc, torn muscles and ligaments, or an out-of-place vertebra in the spine) was the problem that needed to be fixed with medical intervention. Such an explanation would make sense to most medical professionals because a specific mechanical problem can usually be seen with some type of medical exam, such as an MRI or x-ray. Once a doctor can see the image of a specific problem, there are a number of recommended procedures that can "fix" the problem. This is the approach of standard medical treatment for chronic pain.

What was not considered by David's healthcare team was that his pain problem may not be solely a mechanical problem with out-of-place discs, bones, or joints. Rather, his problem may be due to his entire nervous system. We are complex biological, psychological, and social beings, and problems in any area of our lives can impact our entire nervous system and overall health. Only by looking at all the dimensions of who we are

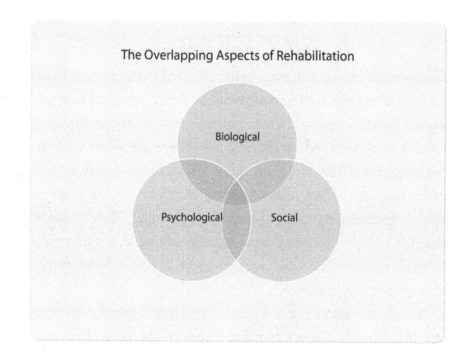

The Overlapping Aspects of Rehabilitation

Biological

Psychological

Social

will we be able to recognize what is out of balance and find a path that moves a person toward health and away from the problems that cause the symptoms of chronic pain.

David and his medical team probably did not know that his chronic pain has something to do with the condition of his central nervous system (the brain and spinal cord). Over time, David's brain and spinal cord have become highly sensitive to the information that they receive from the body, meaning even normal physical movements, or even a light touch, will register in the brain as a threat. When the brain senses a threat, it will produce pain in order to protect against further injury. There were two important questions that no one was asking when David received his previous medical treatment: (1) How did David's central nervous system become overly sensitive? (2) How can David learn to turn down the sensitivity of his central nervous system?

PAIN SCIENCE

The approach to pain management presented in this book is based on expanding research in neuroscience about how the brain and nervous system operate. One component of this research that's central to understanding chronic pain is the discovery that the brain can rewire itself. This is called *neuroplasticity*. The old way of looking at the brain was to view each part of the brain as having specialized functions that never changed. Now we know that the brain is not like a rigid machine. Instead, it's more like a living garden that continues to grow, change, and develop throughout our lives.

The second area of neuroscience that we will rely on throughout this book is the relationship between the central nervous system and pain. The brain and spinal cord have much more to do with our pain than was previously thought. The old way of thinking was narrow, identifying nerve endings and the site of injuries as the main sources of chronic pain. Based on this view, treatments were always focused on stopping the pain at what was believed to be the source of the pain—the lower back, knee, or some other specific spot in the body.

The new science on how the brain and spinal cord operate has radically changed our understanding of pain, helping us understand that the entire central nervous system can become sensitized to pain so that the brain is constantly producing a pain signal, regardless of what healing has already occurred at the site of the injury. *Central sensitization* means that the brain and spinal cord have become overly reactive and sensitive to both normal information, such as a light touch, and to sensations they receive from damage to the body, such as a cut finger or swollen joint.

The third area of science that is central to the approach presented here relates to the *mind-body connection*. The central nervous system (brain and spinal cord) and our immune system are directly influenced by our life experiences. Our experience of pain is not just related to what is happening with our nerve endings or tissue damage. Other events in our lives, past and present, can trigger a stress response.

When our immune response is used to fight off an infection, we benefit from this amazing protective system. Unfortunately, the immune system is not just turned on when we have an infection or a virus. Stress can activate the immune system, and our immune response can do serious damage throughout the body by inflaming joints, tendons, blood vessels, muscles, tissue, and bones. By understanding the mind-body connection, we can see that our thinking, emotions, behavior, and life experiences have a great deal to do with how even a relatively minor injury can eventually develop into a chronic pain problem.

MAKING SENSE OF SCIENCE

The problem with the new knowledge about chronic pain is that it's mostly staying within the scientific community and is not getting to the medical offices, factory floors, retail stores, football fields, offices, and homes of people who live with chronic pain. Let's not wait any longer to dive into this amazing new science. As we begin, the first barrier that many people have is understanding the scientific language often used to describe chronic pain. For example, imagine needing to understand this scientific statement as a starting point for pain education: "Pain relief begins with the simple understanding that peripheral inputs from the Alpha, Delta, and C fibers, and also the Alpha-Beta mechanoreceptor fibers of injured and adjacent non-injured tissues, increase summation of action potentials at the dorsal root ganglion."[1., 2.] While this statement is meaningful to scientists and healthcare professionals, it might not make sense to a person in chronic pain.

While working with patients, attending scientific conferences, reading research articles, and seeing daily news headlines about chronic pain and the opioid epidemic, I realized that what scientists already know about chronic pain and effective pain management is not widely known by healthcare professionals. If most healthcare professionals do not know this information, then the vast majority of the one hundred million chronic pain sufferers in the United States will not know it either.

I want this book to serve as a translation of complicated scientific and medical information into everyday language that the great people I help in the pain rehabilitation program can understand. I want the science of chronic pain to make sense to young and old alike, and to help my healthcare colleagues learn about effective alternatives to pain management that do not involve the standard overused and misused medical interventions.

SKEPTICS WELCOME

I could write a separate book solely about all the skeptical chronic pain patients I have seen. I completely understand their doubts. Some have had over twenty surgeries, all at the recommendation of their doctors who claimed the next surgery would be the final fix they need. Others have had two dozen medications prescribed to them by healthcare professionals who started off treating pain with just one medication but added more to counter side effects caused by the medication. Pain medications can shut down the digestive system, impair the absorption of food and nutrition in the gut, change blood pressure, damage the kidneys, harm the liver, alter brain chemistry, destabilize the mood, and alter memory and thinking. Of course, there are other medications recommended to manage all these unwanted side effects, but they, too, have potential risks and problems. If one pain medication makes you tired and unable to think, then all you need is a good stimulant to keep you awake. But if you are taking a stimulant, then you may also be unable to sleep, have headaches, and increased blood pressure.

It's no surprise that someone who has been through twenty surgeries or has been prescribed twenty-four medications would have some doubts when sitting down in my office for that first consultation. Few are filled with hope and eager anticipation to get help. Most are skeptical and some are angry with the entire healthcare system.

After the first consultation and evaluation, I often hear the question, "You know, I am not so sure about this. I have been treated for pain before and promised improvement and relief that never came. Now I am talking to you, a psychologist. I do not see the point of meeting with you. I have a problem with my neck from a car accident. I do not understand how physical therapy, occupational therapy, and talking with a psychologist is going to do anything about the problem in my neck. My neck was broken, it has screws and rods in it now, and that is not going to change. How are you going to help?"

It is at this point I express how much I appreciate their honesty and welcome their questions and skepticism. What I enjoy about my work is seeing the impact of experience on people's attitudes and beliefs about the possibility of change. During the pain program, patients gradually begin to get off some of the medications that have impaired their thinking. Their ability to concentrate, remember, and problem solving improves. They start moving, stretching, and walking a few minutes at a time. Some begin to sleep longer than two or three hours for the first time in many years. These small changes gradually build hope and undermine their skepticism.

Many people with chronic pain have never met another person with their same type of pain condition, and almost no one has met another pain sufferer who has made a remarkable recovery. For me to give encouragement and hope to chronic pain patients is fine, but I lack credibility. When someone who has suffered from chronic pain for ten years or twenty years gives encouragement and hope to a person just starting the program, that is another matter. Only another pain sufferer knows what another pain patient is going through. Only another fellow pain patient can say, "I have been where you are. I had all the surgeries, injections, and medications. I did not sleep well for years. I do not know how to explain what has changed, but I am moving again, sleeping better, coming off my medications, and doing the things that are important to me. I never thought that this was possible."

Whether you are open, curious, skeptical, angry, depressed, or have already given up, reading this book will give you a different way to look at chronic pain and pain management. Be open to the idea that there might be something in this book that is helpful. While you are reading, share what you are learning with someone else, and maybe you can be a source of hope and freedom for them as well.

2

• • •

CHRONIC PAIN EXPLAINED

There is no single treatment method that will help every person with chronic pain. Before trying to reduce pain, it is important to first understand the principles behind how the brain and body produce pain. To get started, let's take a look at acute pain and see how the mechanisms involved relate to chronic pain. From there, we can start to develop some principles that will be important to know for treating chronic pain.

WHAT IS ACUTE PAIN?

Acute pain is short-acting pain—it can last for just a few minutes or for several weeks. With time, the body heals, and you feel better. If you step on a nail, it is going to hurt. We have a clear understanding of how acute pain like this operates in our brain and body. Tissue damage is registered by specialized nerves in a huge network that runs throughout our entire body. This is the peripheral nervous system. These nerves send information to the spinal cord and brain, which together make up the central nervous system. When there is damage registered by the peripheral nerves, the brain keeps track of where that damage signal comes from.

The central nervous system is always communicating with the peripheral nervous system that runs throughout the body. We have forty-three miles of peripheral nerves that help keep track of balance, temperature, pressure, movement, and damage. The signals between the peripheral nerves and the central nervous system are like wires with a constant flow of electricity running through them. This constant flow of electricity allows the brain to monitor every square inch of the body all at once.

Let's look at what happens when we have an injury. If you accidentally step on something sharp, like a tack or a nail, the electrical activity between the central nervous system and the injured foot increases greatly. When this activity reaches a high intensity, the brain will trigger a pain alarm. The pain alarm is designed to go off only when we are in danger and need protection. Stepping on a nail would be a good example of needing protection. The brain does not want us walking around with a nail in our foot or putting pressure on the foot once the nail is taken out. The brain will also respond by producing a stress response that impacts the entire body and will cause us to walk differently until healing occurs.

Immediately after an acute injury, the electrical activity between the central nervous system and the peripheral nervous system will remain much higher. Because of the increased activity of the nervous system, any small amount of movement, pressure, or vibration will increase the activity just enough to set the pain alarm off again. This is the brain's way of making sure you stay off your foot, protect it, and stay reminded that you need to promote healing.

Since healing tissue damage occurs over several weeks, the electrical communication between the foot and brain eventually decreases. The brain does not need to keep providing the foot with a high level of supervision and protection. When a foot has been punctured by a tack or nail, the central nervous system and peripheral nervous system in the foot will get back to normal levels of communication and electrical activity after several days, so the extreme sensitivity dissipates. You will be able to run and jump as if you never had an injury to your foot.

WHAT IS CHRONIC PAIN?

The explanation of acute pain helps us understand a little about how our entire nervous system works. However, the explanation of acute pain cannot fully explain chronic pain, but it does help.

About 25 percent of people who have acute pain from an injury will end up developing chronic pain. Chronic pain occurs when the sensitivity of the nervous system remains at a high level, even after an injury is healed. Using our previous example, imagine that the electrical activity between the brain and the peripheral nerves in the foot remains elevated after several days. With increased electrical activity, the foot remains sensitive, even though the foot is healing and will eventually heal completely.

Now, why does this sensitivity remain high for some people and not others? To understand chronic pain, we need to understand that our experience of pain involves more than just what happens to our nerve endings. Our experience of pain, both acute and chronic, is influenced by many different factors. Picture a football player with 250 pounds (113 kg) of muscle playing on the football field. Eight other players of equal size run after him, tackling him to the ground. Did getting tackled hurt? Not really. He loves the game and sees soreness as a sign of his toughness

Now picture this same strong player going for his annual sports physical and flu shot before the season begins. A nurse with a tiny syringe walks toward the 250-pound football player waiting for his shot. He slumps to the floor, passed out cold upon seeing the needle. He would tell you he passed out because of the anticipated pain. He just knows it is going to hurt. This response to future pain is based on memory, and these kinds of reactions can help us see how chronic pain develops.

The entire first section of this book is focused on all the factors that influence our perception of pain and how chronic pain develops. For the present moment, we will focus on just three important factors that influence the development of chronic pain: (1) past learning, (2) fear, and (3) evaluating a threat.

PAST LEARNING AND CHRONIC PAIN

Ivan Pavlov (1849–1936) was a Russian physiologist who made an accidental discovery while studying the digestive functions of dogs. When his laboratory assistants brought food for the dogs, the dogs would salivate. Nothing unusual there. Then Pavlov noticed that even when the lab assistants arrived without food, the dogs would still salivate. To understand what was happening, he conducted a simple experiment.

Pavlov gave the dogs food and rang a small bell as they received their food. Day after day, the dogs would get their meal, a bell would ring, and the dogs would salivate. After this routine was established, Pavlov rang the bell but did not bring the dogs food. Just as he expected, the dogs still salivated. The bell and physical response of salivation were paired through *classical conditioning*. The entire process looked like this:

- Food (the stimulus) leads to salivation (the unconditioned response).
- The food is given, and the bell (the neutral stimulus) is rung, which leads to salivation. Pairing the sound of the bell to salivation is called conditioning.
- The food is removed, but the bell alone still leads to salivation (the conditioned response).

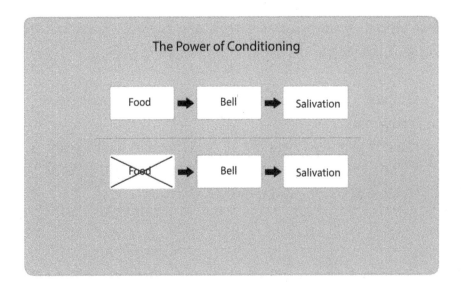

The process that Pavlov discovered is very helpful in explaining how chronic pain can develop. Using the principles of classical conditioning, let's look at how a surgery gone wrong can lead to the development of chronic pain.

In preparation for surgery, Caleb was given an epidural—an injection into his spinal cord with a medication to numb the lower half of his body during the surgery. After the surgery, it was discovered that a hole was left in his spinal cord, causing him to lose spinal cord fluid, called cerebrospinal fluid (CSF). The loss of CSF caused excruciating pain. Caleb had to lay flat on his back and could not lift his head until the hole was repaired. For six months, the hole in his spinal cord could not be fixed, and during that time, Caleb experienced extreme pain with any type of movement.

Finally, after several surgical attempts, the hole was repaired in his spinal cord, and his CSF levels returned to normal in his spine and brain. Problem fixed, right? Not at all. What remained was chronic pain associated with any type of movement he made. Let's look at the classical conditioning steps:

- Injury (the stimulus) leads to pain (the unconditioned response).
- Injury plus movement (the neutral stimulus) leads to pain.
- The injury is removed, but the movement still leads to pain (the conditioned response).

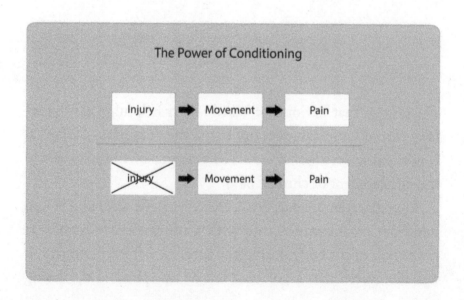

While Caleb was lying flat on his back in bed with a hole in his spinal cord, every lift of his head, roll to his side, or use of the bathroom was associated with agonizing pain. The brain learned very quickly that normal movements, small movements—any movements at all—are linked to pain. This connection in the brain is not something that is just "psychological" or "mental"; the connection is put into the brain's programming software. Learning makes physical changes in the brain, causing different neurons in the brain to become wired together.

The moment Caleb's body was healed of its CSF problem, nothing changed the link his brain had already made between pain and movement. Due to classical conditioning, he continued to have extreme pain with any movement he made. The links in his brain between pain and movement were still firmly in place. Simply put, chronic pain involves a software problem in the brain. The good news is the brain can be reprogrammed.

FEAR AND CHRONIC PAIN

Diabetics get a crash course in pain education, especially children with type 1 diabetes. Imagine how an eleven-year-old boy learns to give himself daily shots. A nurse would have sat down with him and given him an orange and a syringe. Then he would have to start practicing poking the needle into the orange. The nurse would then say something like, "Now you are going to take that needle, fill it with insulin, and poke it right into your stomach. You have to accept that this is what you are going to do for the rest of your life. You are going to start right now with your first injection." Talk about learning pain education the hard way! Then again, maybe this is the easy way because by learning to accept pain and practicing repeatedly over time, he avoids having issues with pain associated with needles.

We can assume the football player who passed out from seeing a needle did not have the advantage of learning to accept this kind of pain. Instead, maybe every time he was given a shot as a child, his mother cried, or someone told him, "This is really going to hurt!" When a person has a strong fear of pain, he or she likely learned that fear from previous experiences. Most people do not recall how they learned their fears, but it is not necessary to recall how fear was learned in order to unlearn it.

Pain is stressful. As we will explore in great detail in this book, when our stress response is activated, we experience even more pain. Fear adds fuel to the fires of stress and pain. Fear is increased when we focus all our attention on concerns like:

- What might happen because of my injury?
- What if I need surgery?
- Will I be able to walk again?
- What if I lose my job?
- What if movement makes my pain worse?
- What if my treatment fails?
- What if I reinjure myself?
- I could lose my house.

We know that regular focus on these concerns will lead to ongoing, heightened sensitivity of the entire nervous system. Fear keeps the connections between the central nervous system and the site of the injury overly active. With the increased electrical activity, any amount of activity or movement, small or large, will trigger the pain alarm. The good news is that a person can learn to overcome fears associated with pain and reduce the overactivity of their nervous system.

EVALUATING A THREAT

Picture a courtroom with a judge and two lawyers. One lawyer provides evidence that the defendant is guilty, and the other lawyer provides evidence that the defendant is innocent. The judge is like our brain. Our brain is constantly gathering evidence about threats to our well-being. If there is enough evidence for the brain to decide that there is a serious threat, it will turn on the pain alarm. On the other hand, if the evidence shows that there is a reason to believe that a person is safe, then the brain will not turn on the pain alarm. Lorimer Moseley, a pain neuroscientist, stated, "A person will experience pain when the credible evidence of threat to the body exceeds the credible evidence of safety to the body."[1.]

Imagine asking people with chronic pain, "How do you know you have chronic pain?" When they answer, they will list all the credible evidence about why they should be in the pain they are in, just like a lawyer in a courtroom. They will list their latest MRI findings, the fact that powerful pain medications and opioids do not help their terrible pain, that all movement is painful, and that their doctor told them they have degenerative disc disease. All of these statements are evidence of a real threat to one's well-being.

When people have chronic pain, the credible evidence they have for safety is weak. They have few reasons to believe that they should not be in chronic pain, few reasons to believe that they could move more without doing harm to themselves, and few reasons for hope that they could get better. One of the benefits of pain education is it increases understanding of how pain actually works, providing a body of knowledge that can strengthen the evidence for safety.

Where are you supposed to get evidence for safety when you are convinced that your MRI, x-ray, or statements from the doctor "prove" you are going to have a life sentence of chronic pain? Patients often feel condemned to a life of chronic pain thanks to statements made by doctors about their medical test results. Patients also think that still having pain after taking powerful pain medications is proof that they have serious chronic pain and that pain cannot be managed. They do not realize their medications may be making their chronic pain worse.

PAIN IS NOT RELATED TO DEGREE OF INJURY

Daniel Clauw is a rheumatologist and professor of anesthesiology, rheumatology, and psychiatry at the University of Michigan and the director of the Chronic Pain and Fatigue Research Center. When Dr. Clauw gives a public lecture on chronic pain, he often starts by showing a picture of two different knee joint x-rays. One knee is healthy and has plenty of cartilage protecting the joint. The other knee has no sign of the protective cartilage, so any movement of the joint will involve "bone on bone."

When doctors explain to their patients the images from MRIs, CT scans, or x-rays, they might say something like this: "You have bone-on-bone damage here. I am surprised you can even walk." Hearing something like this pretty much settles the matter in our minds—we are going to be stuck in pain. But is this really true? What is the evidence that people who have problems like arthritis, pinched nerves, slipped discs, or bone-on-bone joints actually experience pain? The evidence is not very good.

As Dr. Clauw reminds his audiences during his lectures, up to 40 percent of people who have bone-on-bone joint problems experience no pain at all.[2.] The deteriorated joint, for some people, does not lead to reported pain or problems with movement. Not only does a bad knee not always result in pain, but people who have good knees can also have chronic pain. About 10 percent of people who report severe knee pain have no evidence of any inflammation or deterioration.

If knee pain is only caused by the deterioration of the joint, such as the bone-on-bone problem, then it would make sense that medical intervention would help relieve the pain. But it turns out that the standard treatments to relieve this kind of bone-on-bone joint pain, whether surgery or medication, do not reliably lead to reduced pain.[3.] Fortunately, a great deal can be done to help change how the brain is wired, which can change how the brain produces pain. Changing how the brain is wired is also very helpful for those who have knee pain but no sign of injury. Pain, regardless of what is happening in a person's knee, occurs when there is greater evidence of danger than there is evidence for safety. We can change how the brain evaluates what is happening and, as a result, reduce the amount of pain a person experiences.

3

• • •

MISCONCEPTIONS ABOUT PAIN

Pain is strange. Many people have chronic pain without any hard evidence of having a physical injury. Others have had injuries that should have healed, but the pain persists. Headaches and migraines come and go without any indication of what is wrong. In situations like these, pain sufferers are often told by friends, family, and healthcare professionals, "It is all in your head." If you have been given anxiety medication to help manage your pain, your doctor may believe that your pain is not real.

If you or others around you doubt that your pain is real, keep reading. You will learn that pain results from many different factors, some of which we can change, and some we have little control over. All pain is real.

MISCONCEPTION ONE:
PAIN INTENSITY IS RELATED TO THE INJURY

A typical incorrect belief we have of pain is that there is a relationship between what is happening to us physically and the amount of pain we are experiencing. If we poke ourselves with a small straight pin, we might experience a little pain. But if we are using a hammer and accidentally smash our thumb, we assume that we will have a great deal of pain. These assumptions make sense, but they are not always true. What you are going to learn throughout this book is that the commonsense ideas we have about pain are not always correct or true and do not explain chronic pain.

We can experience a lot of pain from very small events, like a paper cut or maybe a small sliver of wood. These events are not much different than a poke from a straight pin, but they can generate a great deal of pain. Small events may lead to a lot of pain or very little pain. It really does not depend on what the event is; pain can be strong, medium, or weak.

What about the hammer? Think of a middle-aged man who works at a desk all day and occasionally needs to do some repairs on his house. When he hits his thumb with a hammer, it hurts. He puts down the hammer, looks for a bag of ice, takes some ibuprofen, complains about his pain, and stops working for twenty minutes.

Now picture a professional carpenter who frames houses for a living. This tradesman will hit his thumb with a hammer, give his hand a shake, say a colorful word or two, and keep working. Within a minute or two, whatever pain he felt is now a distant memory. The tradesman and the do-it-yourself home repairman suffer the same tissue damage, but the tradesman will experience less pain.

It turns out that there is actually no reliable, predictable relationship between what happens to us and the pain we experience. There are many possibilities of what could happen to us and the amount of pain we might feel:

- A minor problem or injury can lead to a little pain.
- A minor problem or injury can lead to no pain.
- A minor problem or injury can lead to a lot of pain.
- A major problem or injury can lead to a little pain.
- A major problem or injury can lead to no pain.
- A major problem or injury can lead to a lot of pain.
- No event or injury can lead to a little pain.
- No event or injury can lead to a lot of pain.

There is no reliable, predictable relationship between what happens to a person and how much pain they experience. This reality poses a significant problem for our traditional ways of thinking about pain, but it is not a problem for the new understanding of how pain works that we have available to us today.

As we explain how pain operates, we will see examples of the many different relationships between what happens due to an injury and what we actually end up sensing as pain. We will discuss why a football player can keep playing with a broken leg and not know it, or why when a mother gives birth and holds her healthy newborn, her lingering childbirth pain will be much different than the mother who sees her baby rushed from the delivery room to receive life-saving surgery. We will even learn how a person who has lost a hand or a leg can experience extreme pain in a missing limb. We do not need nerves for pain, only the brain.

MISCONCEPTION TWO:
PAIN OCCURS IN THE NERVES THEMSELVES

Pain does not occur in the nerves, even when you poke your finger with a pin. When I suggest to my patients that pain is not "in the nerves," they become very interested. Some even ask, "If my pain is not in the nerves, then where is it?" This is just the kind of question that helps pain sufferers become curious and ready to learn.

We have different types of nerve endings that run throughout our body, gathering information and sending it back to the brain for processing. Some of the nerves are specifically dedicated to looking for problems, like a cut or burn. Other nerves are not concerned about problems but are focused on providing the brain with general sensory information, like what the arm of the chair feels like as our fingers run across the surface. These sensory nerves give the brain basic information about vibration, pressure, and touch. All of this information helps the brain keep us safe and explain what is happening around us. The nerves that are specialized in looking for problems come in five different types:

- Nerves focused on tissue damage, such as a cut, scrape, tear, or stretching of tissue.
- Nerves focused on damage from heat, such as picking up a hot cup.
- Nerves focused on mechanical pressure, such as vertebrae in the spine putting pressure on a nerve.
- Nerves focused on chemical detection, such as noticing if we touch acid.
- Nerves focused on inflammation, such as the inflammation of a joint or muscle due to an injury or illness.

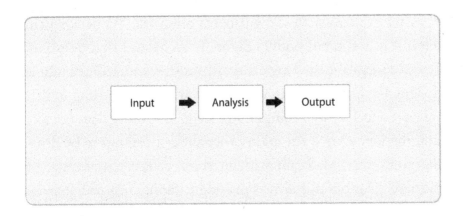

You will often hear these types of nerve endings referred to as "pain nerves," but that description of the nerves is not quite correct. These five types of nerve endings detect change. That is all that they do. They notice that something has changed and respond quickly for our own safety. Simply put, they do not actually detect pain. We do not feel pain in our fingers when we poke ourselves with a pin; we feel pain after the brain has analyzed the information from the tissue nerve in the finger and then produces the sensation of pain. This pain sensation, though perceived as occurring in the finger, comes from the brain.

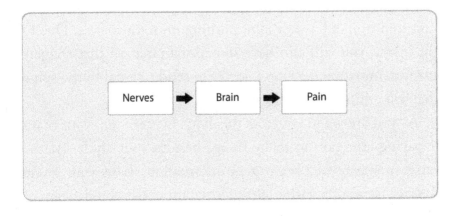

After explaining this, my patients often ask, "Where is pain felt if it is not in our body?" Before I can answer that question, I need to explain the two main tasks of the brain. Our brain is designed to help protect us and explain what is happening so that we have a feeling that things make sense. The brain does not like information, events, sensations, thoughts, or feelings to be floating around in our brain without some category, meaning, or purpose. Our brain is always making meaning or making sense of things, even if the way it organizes information is not correct.

DETERMINING THE GREATEST THREAT

Imagine that you are walking across a busy intersection in Sao Paulo, Brazil. There are five lanes of traffic you have to get across using a pedestrian crosswalk. There is a large group of people that take off with you at the same moment the pedestrian traffic light turns green.

A few steps into the journey, you stumble a little bit, just enough to roll your ankle. The moment you roll your ankle, the spine gets information from the nerves in your ankle with information about tissue damage from a pulled or torn ligament. There might also be some type of mechanical pressure that occurred from a bone or joint pushing on some nerves. Due to the injury, you will also have some inflammation that triggers the inflammation detection nerves to send a signal to the spine that something has changed.

As you are walking across this huge intersection, your brain is paying attention to many things besides your ankle. At the same moment your brain gets information about your ankle damage, it also is gathering information about the dangers of crossing all the lanes of traffic. Your brain is not just concerned that there is a problem in your ankle—it is more concerned with keeping you alive. Because there is a threat to your life as you cross the road, your brain decides to ignore the information sent to it that something has changed with your ankle.

We can imagine the brain saying something like this, "In about five seconds, that traffic light is going to turn red and there will be five large trucks, six taxis, and a dozen motorcycles heading this way. If the body that I am in charge of is standing here thinking about that injured ankle, it's going to get run over. So, for right now, I am *not* going to produce any pain for that ankle, and I will make sure the body gets safely to the other side, out of life-threatening danger." As a result of this brain analysis, you end up walking relatively pain-free to the other side of the road. You take a deep breath, relieved you made it safely.

Suddenly, your brain does a new analysis of the situation. "The person I am in charge of is now out of harm's way. Her life is not in danger, but she should not be walking with all her weight on that ankle. I will make sure she does not injure that ankle any more than it is. I will protect her by producing a good amount of pain so she really pays attention." The next thing you know, the pain in your ankle is sharp and throbbing. You hobble on your painful ankle, being careful to put as little weight as possible on it as you walk.

Now picture one more scene in this story. You are walking down the sidewalk, hobbling on your sore, swollen ankle, and you hear people yelling and screaming behind you. You turn and look and see that a large Bengal tiger has broken loose from the local zoo and is racing down the street right toward you. Your brain will conveniently turn off the pain signal to your ankle, and you will run like a world-class athlete with your sprained ankle until you are safe.

It turns out that our experience of pain is a result of the analysis done by the brain to determine if there is a threat. If the brain determines that there is a threat to your well-being, it will get your attention. The purpose of pain is to protect us from what the brain thinks is a threat of some kind, but the brain will turn on and off the pain depending on what else is going on.

MISCONCEPTION THREE: PAIN IS OUR ONLY WARNING SIGN THAT SOMETHING IS WRONG

Pain is only one of the options that the brain has to get our attention and warn us that something is amiss. Consider what happens if a person has no ability to feel physical sensations due to some type of damage to the spine. Imagine a middle-aged man who fell from a bicycle and was left paralyzed from the middle of his chest down to his feet. He is both unable to move his legs or feel sensations in his lower body. Even when a person experiences such a life-changing event, the brain is still able to monitor and protect a person who is paralyzed.

In the morning, this man goes through his daily routine, including being dressed by a caretaker. When he is being helped with his shoes, the caretaker ties the shoes onto his feet with a normal bow-tie knot. But this particular morning, the knot is tied too tightly. However, due to his spinal cord injury, the man is not able to feel his feet losing circulation from shoes that are too tight. If he did not have the spinal injury, he would first feel the tightness and eventually pain.

The brain needs to bring the problem of the tight shoes to his awareness. Fortunately, the brain has other monitoring systems besides sensory nerves, such as chemical messengers that tell the brain about infections and blood flow. When the brain receives the warning that something is wrong with circulation, it will act. The first thing that this man might notice is that his stomach is upset. All of a sudden, he feels nauseated, queasy, and begins to wonder if he is getting sick with the stomach flu. This is the brain's first attempt to get his attention. If he does not get the message from his brain that something is wrong, the brain will use a different method to get his attention. He will begin to have a painful headache that seems to have come on quickly. Once again, the man assumes that the discomfort he is feeling is related to an illness or stress—he does not recognize that he needs to look over his body for possible problems.

Finally, the brain becomes very determined to let the man know that he is losing circulation in his feet. The brain says, "This guy is not going to be able to see. Let's turn off his vision and make it hard for him to focus his eyes. Next, we will make him throw up anything he has in his stomach. That should do it." If this man has been educated about his condition after his spinal cord injury, he will realize that his brain is desperate to tell him that something is wrong with his body the moment he starts throwing up his breakfast.

With all the brain's warning alarms going off, he gets help from a caretaker, who begins to look for anything that might be wrong with paralyzed areas of his body. When his shoes are untied, the upset stomach, vision problems, headache, and feeling of being sick disappears. The pain leaves because the brain is satisfied that the threat has been taken care of.

HOW THE BRAIN PRODUCES PAIN

Pain begins with input from the nerves, followed by the brain's analysis of the input, which results in output by the brain. First, there is input to the nervous system. There is a muscle strain, a tearing tendon, pressure on a nerve, or inflammation somewhere in the body. This information heads to the spine and then up to the brain, where the brain analyzes that information and makes a determination if there is a threat or not.

If the brain determines there is a threat, then the brain does something to get our attention. The brain could create hives on your face, make your back itch, turn your skin red, make your stomach feel upset, give you a headache, make some part of your body numb, or produce mild, moderate, or severe pain. The brain could very easily do all of these at once if it was that important to pay attention quickly.

Learning to manage chronic pain becomes much easier when we realize that the place where change needs to take place is in the brain and how the software of the brain is working. We cannot change many of the physical problems people have, but we can change how the brain operates and produces pain.

4

• • •

HOW THE BRAIN
ANALYZES PROBLEMS

The key to understanding chronic pain is recognizing the role the brain plays in analyzing all the information it receives from moment to moment from the sensory nervous system spread throughout the body. This analysis is done in a fraction of a second and is generally not something we recognize as happening. As we learn more about what happens in the brain, we'll see how to change how the brain analyzes the information it receives, thereby changing the results of its analyses and leading to a calming of the entire central nervous system. This is how you can achieve improved pain management.

There are three elements of how pain is produced: (1) input from the nervous system indicating something has changed; (2) analysis of the input by the brain to decide if the changes are a threat or not; and (3) output based on the brain's analysis, often the sensation of pain if the brain decided there is evidence of a threat. The key to managing pain is understanding how the brain determines if there is a threat. The brain receives information from the sensory, motor, emotional, cognitive, and behavioral parts of the nervous system and organizes this information into a map—something scientists refer to as a neuromatrix. This chapter will review some of the pieces of the neuromatrix and demonstrate how the brain produces pain when it has determined there is evidence of a threat. By increasing our knowledge of these processes, we can reprogram our brains so they are not always on high alert, protecting us from movements and sensations that are not worthy of a pain sensation.

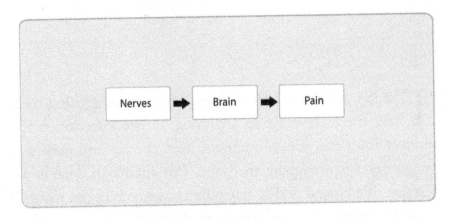

The brain is expertly designed to protect us from problems and to explain or make sense of what is happening. The protecting and explaining aspects of the brain are both essential for our survival and well-being, but they also cause the problems we have with chronic pain. Let's look at the nine processes involved in how the brain analyzes sensory input to see how the goals of explaining and protecting can become connected to chronic pain.

1. LABEL

Our nerve endings each produce a certain quality of sensation that is registered in the brain. Tissue damage from a cut leads to a sharp sensation, while touching a hot surface produces a burning sensation. We feel these different qualities immediately with acute pain. With chronic pain, however, we might experience a range of sensations.

The brain labels the type of sensory experience it detects to help determine how it should respond. The labels used by the brain include sharpness, aching, throbbing, burning, stinging, pulling, electric shock, numbness, tingling, hot, cold, pressure, biting, and dullness. Each of these sensations could be triggered by one or more of the five nerves that detect change. In a general sense, the brain gets an idea of the type of threat from the type of sensation detected. For example, if you have a sharp sensation accompanied by pressure coming from the bottom of your foot, you probably have something in your shoe that needs to be removed so you can walk comfortably.

2. MEMORY

Any information coming into the brain, not just sensory information, is compared with what the brain already knows. Every time you pick up a pencil, the brain does not need to do an in-depth analysis to determine how to hold it, what it is made out of, and how it might be used. All that needs to be done is a simple search of the brain's memory files to see if the pencil is familiar. A quick search comes up with a picture in the memory files that matches the pencil you are seeing sitting on a desk. This process saves time and often saves our lives; we do not have to figure out repeatedly that things like electric cords can be dangerous. Learning this once is enough.

When a person with chronic pain has a sudden surge of pain across the lower back, the brain pulls up a memory. "This is the same kind of pain you had two weeks ago when you stepped out of your car and twisted your back as you stepped up onto the curb." The brain attempts to link the current experience with some previous experience in order to help explain what is currently happening.

The problem with the brain rummaging through our memory files for past similar experiences is that the explanation and comparison might be completely wrong. The cause of the sensation being experienced now may not be related to any past experiences or events that triggered a similar type of pain.

3. CONNECTION

The moment a sensory experience begins, the brain searches for clues about what might be causing the discomfort. Keep in mind there may not be an external event causing the discomfort, but that's where the brain starts its search. The brain needs to explain what is happening and tries to make sense of our experience, even at the expense of correct or useful information that would better explain the circumstances.

As usual, Christine spends part of her day in the kitchen working on the dirty dishes. After standing at the sink for about fifteen minutes, rinsing breakfast and lunch dishes and putting them into the dishwasher, she experiences lower back pain. It starts as a dull ache with a slight pulling sensation, but it's not long before a sharp pain forces her to stop what she is doing.

As her pain increases, her brain scrambles to make sense of all that is happening. The brain reasons that standing for fifteen minutes has caused her pain. You can picture the brain saying something like, "What was she thinking, standing in one place for so long? Standing is bad for the lower back. This is definitely going to cause problems for the lower back." This is the first connection the brain makes between pain and her current activities.

While standing at the sink, Christine looks out the window above the kitchen sink and sees the weather changing. The blue sky is disappearing, and dark billowy clouds are rolling in. The wind starts picking up, and the temperature begins to drop. Christine realizes a storm is settling in and will probably be there for a while. Once again, the brain sees something that might be useful in explaining what is happening. "Look at the storm! Temperature and barometric pressure changes are going to trigger pain for Christine. That is what always happens." This is the second connection the brain makes between pain and what it thinks is a possible cause.

Now the brain has two clear causes that it can point to and concludes it has done its job at making sense of Christine's pain. But there are problems with this explanation. The first problem is that it "feels right" or at least plausible to Christine, making her not look for any other explanation or evidence. The second and more important problem with the explanation is that it is likely wrong. Her back pain may have nothing to do with standing too long or the change in the weather.

4. PAST LEARNING

In chapter 2, we outlined how the brain can learn to link pain with movement. An injury occurs, and this injury is serious enough to cause pain. While the injured person is recovering, any movement they make produces pain. Over time, movement becomes linked to pain. Once the individual heals from their injury, the brain has learned through classical conditioning that movement and pain are now linked together. Besides movement, other activities, objects, and places can be linked with pain.

5. PREDICTION

Once the brain labels an experience, links it to a specific memory, and generates reasons for the discomfort, it has enough information to make a prediction about how long the discomfort will last. The brain says something like, "The last time Christine had pain like this, she was standing in a grocery store for almost an hour. She was in pain for the rest of the day when that happened. The discomfort she is having now, especially with this bad weather starting up, is going to last for at least eight hours today."

But how does the brain know how long the discomfort is going to last? Well, it doesn't know. The brain cannot accurately predict how long pain will last, but these predictions help the brain come up with a plan to protect the person from additional problems. Even though this planning can be helpful, the problem with the prediction about how long the pain will last is that the brain does not know for sure—it is only guessing. It could last five minutes or five hours.

6. JUDGMENT

Regardless of the cause of pain, illness, or injury, our brain has an interesting way of reframing the events of our lives so that we end up at the center of what happened, especially if what happened is bad. Our brain is designed to protect and explain, but it sometimes doesn't do either of these well when there is a lack of information. If the brain views something harmful as completely outside of our control, we might not learn from what happened or protect ourselves if it happens again. To "correct" for this, the brain will twist the rules of logic and reason and come up with a version of events that ends up feeling like we are to blame for what happened. Many of the patients I have worked with struggle with thoughts like:

- I should be able to stop this pain when it flares up. I am not trying hard enough.
- I should have been in better shape when the accident happened.
- I must not be doing what the doctors have recommended correctly or seriously enough. That is why I am suffering from pain.
- If I was a better person, I would not be suffering from chronic pain.
- I have done things in my life that I am not proud of, and this pain is my payback.

The brain is constantly evaluating and rating thoughts, events, emotions, and memories as good or bad, positive or negative. There is nothing we can do to stop this, but there are things we can do to help notice what the brain is doing so that these judgments are not believed as true or valid.

7. STORY

Once chronic pain becomes a part of your life, how you see your life changes. Rather than seeing yourself in charge of what is happening, pain becomes the author of your story.

Picture yourself on a Monday night receiving a phone call from an old friend. Several former college friends are getting together next Saturday. Then comes the expected question: "So, are you coming?"

You say, "I just don't know."

This does not satisfy your friend. "Why don't you know? Do you have something else planned?" the friend asks.

"No," you reply. "The thing is, I just don't know how I am going to feel on Saturday. You had better call me on Friday. Better yet, call me on Saturday morning. I will probably know how I am going to feel in the morning and hopefully will feel good enough to make it."

Not only does your brain have the ability to predict how long your pain will last during the day, but it also will predict that pain will be the one determining how your life story unfolds.

8. QUESTIONS

In order for the brain to protect and explain, it needs to be able to anticipate problems. Questions are basic to our thinking process; we are constantly evaluating what we are encountering, and a key part of that evaluation is asking questions.

You probably have spoken with your primary care doctor about your chronic pain and received some kind of explanation and treatment suggestions. Then you are referred to an orthopedic specialist, who, after evaluating you, refers to you a neurologist, who refers you to a pain specialist. Now you have seen four doctors and have four different explanations of your pain and different recommendations for pain management. Your brain is going to ask the obvious question: "Does anyone know what they are talking about? I have four different explanations!" These questions can stir up anxiety and fear.

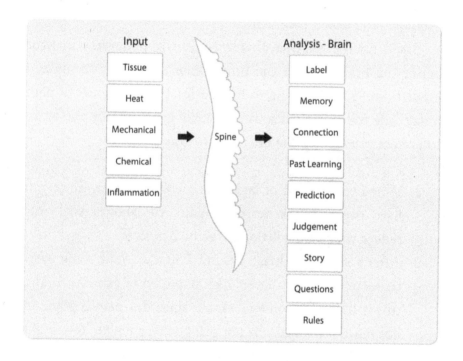

9. RULES

In order for the brain to protect us, it needs to determine what we can and cannot do so that we do not make the problem we have worse. To accomplish this task, the brain creates a wide variety of rules that we need to follow throughout the day to stay on what the brain thinks is a safe path. As with the other activities of the brain listed so far, there is both good and bad to the rules the brain creates to protect us.

The brain creates rules the moment it begins to evaluate the cause of pain. Imagine waking up at 6:00 a.m. and taking an inventory of your body and your night's sleep. As you are lying there, you notice that your back is a bit stiff. Both sides of your neck muscles in the back are aching and a bit sore. Then you have a sharp pain shooting down your neck, over to the left shoulder, and down your arm.

Based on the analysis that was already underway in your brain, the brain has all the information it needed to make a prediction—you are going to have at least twelve hours of pain today. The following rules were quickly generated by the brain to protect you during the next twelve hours:

1. When you get out of bed, take a warm shower. Since you have twelve hours' worth of pain, the shower will only reduce your pain a little, maybe by 2 percent.

2. After you eat breakfast, around 7:30 a.m., take some over-the-counter pain relievers like ibuprofen or aspirin. Again, this will provide some relief, but since this pain is going to last most of the day, it is not going to be enough. You might get a 15 percent reduction in pain from the pain relievers.

3. Around 10:00 a.m., you are going to start hurting a bit more just from the activity of the day. That is when you are going to need to take a prescribed pain reliever. Keep in mind, your pain level is going to be high today. Twelve hours of discomfort is a serious threat to your well-being, so the prescribed medicine may not be enough to give you the relief you need.

4. In order for you to get the best impact from the prescribed medicine, you are going to need to lay down and take a nap around noon. If you sleep for thirty minutes, it might help. But if you don't sleep at all, or worse, you sleep for only five minutes, you are going to be miserable for the rest of the day.

5. Around 4:00 p.m., your pain is still going to be there because this is twelve hours' worth of pain today, so you are going to need another prescribed medication to make it through the rest of the day. Because you will have already taken over-the-counter medication and two doses of the prescribed medication, you are going to be in a brain fog and not be able to think clearly. Therefore, do not plan to do anything, go anywhere, or interact with anyone. You had better cancel all your plans now because you just won't be able to function well enough to enjoy them.

The rules created by your brain are designed to protect you during the predicted twelve hours of pain. The problem with the rules created by the brain is that they are not designed to help you overcome your problem with chronic pain. The rules function to limit activity and reduce stimulation, neither of which is helpful in overcoming chronic pain. If we listen to the rules all the time, we will be protected from pain for short periods of time, but we will not heal. Healing will require breaking the rules our brains are coming up with that are designed only for short-term protection.

In the next chapter, we will add to the analysis and include the role that emotions play in the decision-making process of the brain.

5

OUR BUILT-IN WARNING SYSTEM

Emotions are central to the brain's analysis of how to protect us and explain what is happening, amplifying important themes that emerge. Emotions play a central role in the brain's neuromatrix, which determines if pain needs to be produced. When the brain asks worrisome questions, our emotions intensify those questions and add emotions like anxiety, fear, or sadness. Because of our emotions, we take seriously what the brain is telling us. We do not like negative emotions, and we are highly motivated to get rid of them as fast as possible. Our negative emotions motivate us to change. This is similar to how other systems in the body operate, such as thirst. Thirst is uncomfortable, and we are driven to reduce our thirst by looking for water to drink.

Emotions are similar to our taste buds. When we put something into our mouths, we immediately taste it. If our nose and tongue are working properly, our taste buds will warn us of what is not good to eat, such as sour milk, and inform us what is good to eat, such as freshly baked bread still warm from the oven. Our emotions are similar. By paying attention to what we feel, we can learn a great deal about the problems we face and health issues that deserve our attention. In this chapter, we will look at several emotions that can directly impact our experiences with chronic pain.

1. FEAR

We experience fear when there is a threat to our well-being, usually our physical well-being. A large, angry, barking dog running toward us will trigger fear because the dog represents a potential threat. We might get bitten by this dog, and fear motivates us to do something to avoid this. Fear is unpleasant, and we would rather not have it running throughout our bodies.

When a person is experiencing ongoing problems with pain, fear can easily be triggered by questions such as: Do I have cancer? Is there some kind of tumor that is causing my pain? Will I need surgery? These kinds of questions do not have quick and easy answers. Fear amplifies the seriousness of the questions and motivates us to get answers or find ways to at least reduce the tension caused by the fear.

2. ANXIETY

Anxiety is similar to fear, but anxiety is its own emotion. The key element of anxiety is a lack of control. Picture driving in the winter and you hit a patch of ice on the road. You turn the steering wheel to the right, but nothing happens. You turn to the left, but the car does not change directions. You just keep sliding closer and closer toward oncoming traffic. When driving on ice, you have no control, and the resulting emotion is anxiety.

Anxiety is a very unpleasant emotion, and we are highly motivated to stop it in its tracks. The wish to get rid of anxiety, as we will learn more about later, actually makes the anxiety worse. The value of anxiety is that it motivates us to change our situation and regain some type of control or the perception of control.

We often experience a lack of control when we struggle with chronic pain. One Monday morning, you wake up with a moderate to severe level of pain and say to yourself, "I am going to try to do some new stretches that I have learned recently. Then I will do some exercises with rubber fitness-bands for ten minutes. After that, I will take some ibuprofen to help with the pain." Within one hour of this simple routine, you feel better. Then on Tuesday morning, you wake up with similar pain and say to yourself, "Well, I know what works. I will try my new favorite exercises and stretches to manage pain." But on this particular day, nothing happens. In fact, you end up feeling worse from the exercises and stretches.

When we feel that there is no connection between what we do and the results we get, we experience a loss of control. This also occurs with some chronic pain sufferers who are very active with relatively little pain one day, but then do very little activity and experience a great deal of pain on another day. When the pain comes and when it goes does not seem to make sense. The same goes for what brings relief and what does not. These situations increase our sense of anxiety due to the lack of control over what is happening to us.

3. SADNESS

With the onset of chronic pain, there are going to be losses. Chronic pain interferes with almost every aspect of life. Pain gets in the way of enjoying work, hobbies, using your hands, and socializing with friends or sitting through a church service. Because of pain, the positive parts of life are taken away from a person's normal routine until he or she is left with very little to enjoy. When we experience loss, we experience sadness.

Sadness is an important reminder that parts of our lives that were once rich and meaningful are no longer present. Sadness is easy to identify when we experience the death of a friend or family member, but it can be harder to recognize when it is linked to the losses that come with chronic pain. Often, we are too focused on trying to manage the pain, attend medical appointments, and just survive the next twenty-four hours to notice all the subtle changes that have been taking place.

Because of pain, one enjoyable activity after another is set aside. Saying no to social invitations becomes routine. Weeks of focusing on pain management soon become months, which turn into years. The struggle to get by might distract a person from feeling sad for a period of time, but not forever. Eventually, sadness shows up and brings a heaviness to a person's life. Many of the good things that were once commonplace are now gone, except for the memories.

4. ANGER

Anger is a powerful reminder of unfairness and injustice. You probably have watched on the evening news some type of story about a child being hurt, abandoned, or abused. Your internal response is one of anger. You say to yourself, "That is not fair! That child does not deserve such terrible treatment." When we feel that something is unfair, we are then motivated to do something helpful to set things right. We might give money to a social service agency that helps needy children, or we might decide to get directly involved in helping children by working in an after-school program or providing foster care.

Anger is a valuable emotion that can help us to make right what is wrong. However, we need to be very careful when we feel angry and ensure that our sense of what is right and wrong is correct. It's easy to think things are not fair just because we do not like them. If we are angry about sitting in a traffic jam, we are viewing the traffic jam as if it is unfair to us personally, but it's not.

Anger often occurs with chronic pain because pain interferes with life. We usually picture our lives going in a certain direction, then all of a sudden, an obstacle blocks our path. This obstacle is chronic pain. Pain stops us from being able to go forward with our lives. Imagine going up to the roadblock and asking, "Hey, what's the deal? Why is this here?" The only problem is no one is there to answer your question.

If pain has shown up in your life, you know your life has drastically changed. This may seem unfair, and we can become very angry about how chronic pain has changed the direction our lives were heading.

5. FRUSTRATION

Think of frustration as low-level anger. You are reading a wonderful novel on a warm, lazy afternoon, sitting on a porch swing in the shade. While you are in the best part of the book, a fly starts buzzing near your ear, then in your face, and then it disappears only to return again, this time near your other ear. A fly interrupting your reading seems unfair and leads to frustration but not full-blown anger.

Frustration is one of the most common emotions I hear patients report. With acute pain, the pain level will go from zero up to five and then back down to zero in a few hours. This does not usually happen with chronic pain. Chronic pain starts off at a level two, then goes up to a level six, and finally settles down at a level four. The pain rarely goes away completely. As soon as a chronic pain sufferer is quiet and settled down, the awareness of pain comes back, just like a fly that shows up while reading a good book. This is very frustrating.

6. HELPLESSNESS

We have a basic need to accomplish what is important to us. For example, if we want to prepare a meal for our family, then we need to do all the steps involved to make that happen. If we cannot do all the steps, regardless of how hard we try, we are going to end up feeling helpless.

Chronic pain sufferers frequently receive advice on how to manage pain from healthcare professionals. Rarely does a health-care professional say, "I don't know what to tell you to do about your pain." They always give advice, tips, exercises, suggestions, support devices, medications, and treatment. Chronic pain patients will try all of these suggestions because they are desperate for relief. They want to feel better and hope that the suggestions and advice work. After trying one idea after another, patients begin to feel that the things they are trying are not effective. When no strategy works, a sense of helplessness can weigh on a person every day. Self-judgment can make this feeling of helplessness worse as the brain begins to blame the person for not trying hard enough, not having a strong faith, or giving up too easily.

7. DEPRESSION

Unfortunately, depression is an emotion that is hard for people in our society to talk about openly, even though it is so common that almost everyone will experience it at some point. Feeling helpless about managing pain can often lead to depression. When we are helpless, we cannot make necessary changes in our lives, and giving up this fight is experienced as depression.

The feeling of powerlessness and being ineffective in one area of life can spread to other areas of our lives almost like a virus. Consider the negative thought, "I am ineffective at changing my life to manage my pain." This negative thought is a thought virus. The thought virus "I am powerless" starts off referring to your health. You try to manage your chronic pain but do not succeed. You then try again, this time a bit harder with a new and improved technique. Still no change. But thought viruses, like real physical viruses, do not like to stay in one place; they travel. Your thought virus spreads to other areas of your life. Your thinking begins to change in every dimension of who you are:

- Marriage: I am not a very good spouse. My chronic pain is ruining my marriage, and there is nothing I can do about it.
- Parenting: I am not a very good parent. My kids seem unhappy, and it is probably my fault.
- Work: I am not a very good employee. There are always problems at work, and I just do not handle them well. I am probably making things worse for everyone.
- Hobbies: I am not very skilled at doing things I used to enjoy. I am not sure why this was even a hobby of mine. If I cannot do it well, I should not even bother trying at all.

- Friendships: I am not a very good friend. My friends are probably tired of hearing about my problems and tired of me turning down invitations.
- Future: I am not able to see any good in the future. All I have to look forward to are the same bad things that I am experiencing now.

When we have a negative view of ourselves, a negative view of the future, and a negative view of our circumstances, we are depressed. There are a surprising number of patients whom I have seen over the years who are clearly depressed but do not know it because they do not recognize these basics signs of depression.

When we feel powerless to make important changes in our lives, we are going to experience depression. The key to change is not stopping, masking, or numbing the depressing emotions, but changing the thinking and behavior that feeds the depression. We need to find ways to face the challenges that cause us to feel powerless without letting our sense of helplessness infect every dimension of our lives.

8. SHAME

Shame is the feeling of being defective and negatively judged by others. We might hear others being judgmental, or we may feel judged even when we cannot hear the words being said. A common experience that chronic pain sufferers have is meeting an old friend whom they have not seen in months or years. The friend says, "You are still having chronic pain? You look just fine! You are laughing and smiling—you don't seem like you are in pain. You should drink more herbal tea. That will help you get rid of your pain."

Comments from friends and family increase a pain sufferer's feeling that something is wrong with them. Even physicians can add to this sense of shame by telling a patient their pain is all in their head.

BRAIN ANALYSIS

When an injury occurs, the brain has to determine if that sensory information it receives from the peripheral nervous system indicates a threat. Emotions play a key role in amplifying the analysis the brain is doing and increases the level of threat to the point that pain is produced.

Imagine a fifty-five-year-old man who works in an office all day. He is a bit out of shape—deconditioned, as healthcare professionals like to say. One weekend, he starts to work in his

Input	Analysis	Brain Emotion
Tissue	Label	Fear
Heat	Memory	Anxiety
Mechanical	Connection	Sadness
Chemical	Past Learning	Anger
Inflammation	Prediction	Frustration
	Judgement	Helplessness
	Story	Depression
	Questions	Shame
	Rules	

yard, cutting down trees, moving dirt, and pulling up shrubs. While he is working, his chest muscles become sore. The man ignores his sore chest, and thirty minutes later, his left shoulder begins to hurt.

The brain does some analysis and is uncertain about what is causing the soreness. The brain asks, "Could this soreness be the sign of a heart attack?" This question is not easy to answer, so fear and anxiety are triggered by the brain. When fear and anxiety are triggered, muscle tension increases. In the man's case, the brain becomes convinced that this soreness is not normal, but an actual sign of a heart attack. This increases fear and anxiety, and the brain's threat detector is turned up to its highest level of sensitivity because the brain believes it now has credible evidence for danger. Instantly, intense chest pain is produced. This chest pain, like fear and anxiety, motivates the man to rush to the nearest hospital, only to be told he is not having a heart attack and is simply out of shape.

When the man hears the news that he is not having a heart attack, the brain recalculates the possibility of a threat and determines that there is more credible evidence of safety than there is of danger. The evidence for safety has come from the reassuring words of the doctor. Now the brain views the discomfort in the chest and shoulder as normal soreness and, as a result, turns off the output of pain.

6

● ● ●

STRESS INCREASES CHRONIC PAIN

C hronic pain triggers another protective response in our bodies—the stress response. The stress response can be helpful in some situations, but when a person has chronic pain, the stress response can also become chronic and do more harm than good.

Chronic stress, however, causes changes in the immune system and how the nervous system operates, making the pain worse. Stress is a key factor in creating and maintaining chronic pain.

THE STRESS RESPONSE

Before we focus on how stress can damage the body and increase chronic pain, it is important to first understand how stress impacts the body in the short term. Acute stress lasts for a short period of time, and we recover quickly from all the changes that occur in our brain and body because of it.

Picture yourself riding in a car through a town or city. You travel downtown through the busy intersections and have plenty of other vehicles on the road with you. All of a sudden, from someplace that you cannot see, you hear the screeching of tires on the road. In an instant, your ears give you a lot of information. As the sound travels to your ears, your brain determines that the sound is coming from a heavy vehicle, maybe a large truck, and that the sound is traveling directly to your current position and is now very close. That is all the information you have, but it is enough to start an amazing chain of events within your brain and body.

The acute stress you are experiencing as the truck approaches provides a rough picture of the response that the brain and body go through each time we experience stress, be it acute, chronic, or traumatic. The body and brain can react with varying intensity, but the basic reactions to all stressful events are similar. The body prepares us for one of three possible events: (1) to fight against the possible threat; (2) to run from the threat; or (3) to protect us by shutting down all the normal responses so quickly it stops all movement, which might be helpful for hiding and remaining unnoticed. Because of these three possible actions, we often call this stress response the *fight-flight-freeze response*.

To understand more about how our bodies respond to acute stress, it is helpful to learn how the nervous system automatically keeps track of different bodily processes.

OVERVIEW OF
THE NERVOUS SYSTEM: SIMPLIFIED

To keep the explanation simple, I will start with the easy-to-understand version of how the nervous system works. Our brains keep things running so we do not have to think about our heartbeats, breathing, blood pressure, and staying alert.

These functions and many others throughout the body are controlled automatically. This automatic system has two parts: a gas pedal, which speeds up biological processes; and a brake, which slows things down. Under stress, the gas pedal is applied, and our heart rate, breathing rate, and blood pressure increase, and blood sugar and all kinds of hormones are released.

To keep the stress response from getting out of control, the brake will slow down all the activities of the body and lower the heart rate, breathing rate, and blood pressure. Learning to manage stress involves recognizing when the gas pedal has been pushed and noticing the changes that have occurred in the body. Then, knowing how to put on the brakes can slow down the stress response.

If this simplified version of the nervous system makes sense, and you do not want an additional explanation of everything involved in the stress response, great! Just skip the next section and start reading at "The Impact of Chronic Stress."

OVERVIEW OF
THE NERVOUS SYSTEM: DETAILED

There are two basic parts of the nervous system: the central nervous system, which is the brain and spinal cord; and the peripheral nervous system, which is all the other nerves that run throughout the body. The peripheral nervous system has two divisions as well. One part regulates activities like heart rate, blood pressure, digestion, breathing, salivation, and pupil dilation. This is called the *autonomic nervous system* (ANS) because it runs biological processes automatically. The second part of the peripheral nervous system is the *somatic nervous system*, which controls how our muscles move. The somatic nervous system is largely under our voluntary control. It's what allows me to move my arm when I think about moving it.

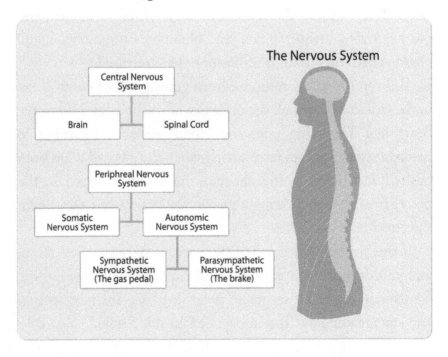

The Nervous System

When our bodies become activated by a stressor, such as the screeching brakes of a truck skidding toward us, our response is controlled by the ANS. The ANS takes information from the brain about a possible threat and prepares the body for action. The ANS has two divisions that work in constant coordination to prepare us for action. The *sympathetic system* prepares us for action by working with our emotions and increasing arousal throughout the body. The *parasympathetic system* works against emotional arousal and relaxes muscles, restores digestion, and helps with healing. These two amazing systems work together every moment of our lives to keep everything in balance. Stress knocks these two systems out of balance.

BRAIN AND BODY CHANGES
FROM ACUTE STRESS

The response of the sympathetic nervous system to a threat starts in the brain and spreads quickly throughout the entire body. A hormone, corticotropin-releasing hormone (CRH), is released in the hypothalamus in the brain, which triggers the pituitary gland, also in the brain, to release a hormone called adrenocorticotropic hormone (ACTH) that travels through the bloodstream and triggers the adrenal glands, on top of the kidneys. The adrenal glands then release hormones that send chemicals, such as adrenaline and cortisol, throughout the body to make many of the stress response changes that help prepare for action.

The obvious, more noticeable changes that happen with the stress response include increased heart rate, increased blood pressure, increased breathing rate, reduced saliva production, increased blood sugar, blood vessel constriction, strengthened muscles, and hormones that help dampen the feeling of pain. Blood circulation also changes so that the hands and feet receive less blood. This helps core muscles become stronger as blood flow to this area increases. This explains why your hands and feet become cold when you are under stress.

Your stomach stops digesting food, and the intestines process food and absorb nutrients slower. Whatever is in your bowels and bladder might be immediately pushed out of your system to reduce weight and free up energy to deal with more important things. Prolactin, a hormone, is also released by the pituitary gland, which has at least two effects. Prolactin helps us manage pain, but it will also interfere with reproduction, which may explain why couples who are experiencing stress are not able to become pregnant. When stress is prolonged, the stomach releases fewer prostaglandins, which protect the stomach from acid needed to digest food. This increases pain in the stomach and can lead to gastroesophageal reflux disease.

THE IMMUNE RESPONSE DURING CHRONIC STRESS

When the stress response activates during acute stress, as will happen when a person is in a car accident, the fight-flight-freeze response is exactly what the body needs to prepare for action. The problem in our modern world, however, is that many of the stressors we face do not involve some type of physical threat. Modern-day stressors show up in the form of upsetting emails, traffic jams, pressure from the work we do every day, and our responsibilities at home.

The body's alarm system is well suited for a physical attack from a bear but not for sitting at a desk and trying to solve an accounting problem for hours. Likewise, the stress response is not completely helpful when dealing with the daily strain experienced by a person with chronic pain. However, it can be helpful to know that stress, like pain, is complicated; it turns out that our stress response is not nearly as damaging to our health as is our view of stress. We will discuss how to view stress later in the book.

The immune system does a fantastic job of protecting us and is directly impacted by acute stress responses. If we are cut or have a broken bone, white blood cells are there to help. But what happens if the body does not have any injury? The white blood cells are still going to be released, and they are going to be coursing through the entire body. When acute stress occurs, the immune system response is helpful, but this is not the case in chronic stress and traumatic stress.

When the body is under chronic stress, two different responses occur throughout the body. First, the normal immune functions of the body are suppressed or kept from working as well as they normally would. With chronic stress, there is an increase in cortisol released by the adrenal glands. When cortisol levels remain high, the immune system is suppressed, preventing it from fighting off infections and viruses. It also increases the likelihood a person will become insulin resistant and develop type 2 diabetes. This is why upsetting events like divorce, unemployment, or even a stressful college exam schedule can make people more vulnerable to the flu, herpes, viral infections, chickenpox, mononucleosis, and the Epstein-Barr virus.[1, 2.] Even people who undergo surgery will recover much more slowly if they were experiencing chronic stress before the surgery.

The second aspect of chronic stress that differs significantly from acute stress is the inflammation response. With chronic stress, cytokines (proteins that send signals to other cells) are released by cells throughout the body. Cytokines have two effects related to chronic pain. First, there are some specific types of cytokines that will increase sensory nerve sensitivity. This means that nerves responsible for identifying problems and change become overly sensitive to anything and everything around them. Second, there are other types of cytokines that cause inflammation. This inflammation can occur anywhere throughout the body, such as in joints, ligaments, tendons, muscles, nerves, blood vessels, the skin, and thyroid glands.

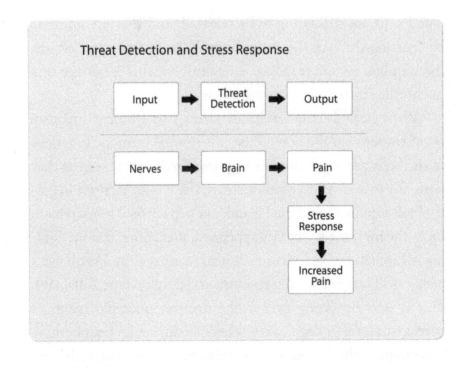

Threat Detection and Stress Response

Chronic stress is associated with heart disease, type 2 diabetes, some types of cancer, lupus, psoriasis, fibromyalgia, arthritis, inflammatory bowel disease, and a number of other autoimmune diseases. Our immune systems are able to help protect us when there is an injury or infection, but when we are under chronic stress, our immune systems can work against us, weakening our ability to fight off infections, increasing pain sensitivity, and increasing inflammation. Autoimmune disorders are increasingly common in the U.S., affecting at least twenty-three million people, a figure that grows by 7 percent every year.[3.] It is not uncommon for chronic pain sufferers to also report having autoimmune conditions such as hives, irritable bowel syndrome, Crohn's disease, dry eyes, dermatitis, hypothyroidism, arthritis, and hair that falls out.

Chronic pain and stress are linked. Chronic pain will increase a person's level of stress, and stress will increase a person's level of chronic pain. In fact, stress is a key contributor to acute pain becoming chronic pain. Unfortunately, we often do not recognize the symptoms of stress or the issues in our lives that add to our stress. Increasing our awareness of what is happening in our mind, body, and relationships will be the focus of the next two sections of the book, which discuss how to calm the nervous system and develop emotional flexibility.

7

• • •

THE IMPACT OF CHRONIC STRESS

Rachel was sitting on the edge of an examination table in the emergency room, waiting to be seen by a nurse and then the physician. She had no idea how this could be happening to her. A few years ago, she developed some numbness in her fingertips. Then over the past year, her hands began to have a strange tingling sensation, and her arms began to ache. After seeing her primary care doctor, she was referred to a neurologist because her doctor thought Rachel might have fibromyalgia. But that was not why she was in the ER now—at this moment, she was convinced she was having a heart attack.

Up until being diagnosed with fibromyalgia two years ago, Rachel had considered herself healthy. She was only thirty-eight years old, watched her diet, and was always busy. Even as a full-time working mother of two young children, she took the time to stay in shape by walking with her children and the family dog every evening. Yet, there was no denying that something was wrong with her as she waited in the emergency room.

She had read that some chronic pain conditions can impact different aspects of the nervous system, even the part of the nervous system that controls the heart. She wondered if that is what was happening to her. The chest pain, sweating, and tightness came out of the blue late one Sunday evening. She was getting her children ready for bed and herself ready for the next morning at the office, where she worked as a manager.

For the medical staff in the emergency department, it was not surprising to see an otherwise healthy thirty-eight-year-old woman like Rachel having heart attack symptoms, in part because cases like this are so common. Even though the medical team had a strong suspicion that Rachel was not having a heart attack, they followed the standard protocol for evaluating Rachel, which included extensive blood work and an EKG to examine the rhythm of her heart.

After a few hours of waiting, the results were in. Rachel did not have a heart attack and was in fact quite healthy, apart from the chronic pain of fibromyalgia. Rachel was relieved at the good news, but she was also confused. How could she be told that she was healthy and at the same time have shortness of breath, a rapid heart rate, chest tightness, intense chest pain, and blurred vision? If that was not a heart attack, what was it?

Like anyone in this situation, Rachel had a lot of questions for her doctor. She did not even know where to begin. "What in the world happened to me? I had sudden chest pain, I could hardly breathe, my left arm went numb, and I was sick to my stomach. I could not even think or see straight. I was sweating as if I had just run a marathon, and I never sweat. I just do not get it."

The physician knew that this question was coming. She has had this conversation with patients many times before, but it was never easy knowing where to begin. She asked Rachel, "Do you have any stress in your life right now?"

This simple question hit Rachel like a terrible accusation. She wondered to herself: "Why in the world is the doctor asking me this? Is she going to say this was all in my head? There is no way this was in my head. I was dying of a heart attack a few hours ago. I know what I went through."

Rachel composed herself and politely asked, "I do not know why you are asking me this question. What does stress have to do with this?"

The doctor was not surprised by her confusion and signs of anger. She responded by repeating her question, "You seem confused about why I am asking you about stress. That is okay. I will answer your question. But for right now, I am wondering if you can tell me a little about your life. What is going on that might be stressful? Have there been any changes, big or small, in your life in the past few months?"

After taking a long breath in, Rachel said, "Well, I am a mother of a six-year-old and eight-year-old. That is stressful all by itself. I work a full-time job as a manager of a large business, but I really like my job. Recently, meeting my career and home responsibilities has become more difficult because of my fibromyalgia. My pain started in my hands and has moved up my arms. Now I am getting pain across my back for some reason. I recently started going to a chiropractor. My husband is a nice guy, but he, too, is working full-time, and we don't seem to have much time for each other. Sometimes I think he is avoiding being home—maybe I am just imagining it. I don't know. So, I really don't know how to answer your question. My life seems pretty normal to me. I obviously do not like the numbness, tingling, and pain that I have in my hands and arms."

The doctor expected this answer. She knew that if Rachel was aware of her stress and how it was impacting her mind and body, she probably would not have ended up in the emergency room. If Rachel recognized what her stress was doing to her, she would have made some changes to how she lived her life.

FACING REALITY

To help Rachel understand stress, the doctor explained, "Rachel, when a person has stress, it is easy to not pay attention to what is happening. We are all vulnerable to the temptation to put difficult life issues on the back burner, telling ourselves that it's not so bad, that others have it worse, and that we have a lot to be thankful for. Meanwhile, the small- and medium-sized stressors start to pile up. Tell me, when did you get your diagnosis of fibromyalgia?"

Rachel sighed. She hated even thinking about that episode in her life. Her primary care doctor was not sure what caused her unusual symptoms and referred her to a rheumatologist. It turned out that this particular rheumatologist did not "believe in" fibromyalgia and seemed irritated that Rachel was even sent to his office. He suggested that Rachel see a neurologist. After she waited two months for the scheduled appointment with the neurologist, Rachel was very angry about seeing this new doctor. Unlike the previous physician, the neurologist completed the standard medical assessment tool for diagnosing fibromyalgia. The neurologist examined Rachel, gathered her history, and then told her that she clearly met the diagnostic criteria for fibromyalgia and then started her on an anticonvulsant medication called Lyrica.

The neurologist suggested that Lyrica (pregabalin) would help her manage her symptoms, but after only a few months of taking the medication, Rachel had gained weight, often felt dizzy, and had a hard time functioning at work because of drowsiness and difficulty focusing her vision while reading. Since she was not tolerating the medication, she was slowly taken off it, which itself was another struggle because the withdrawal made her nauseous and have terrible headaches.

The emergency room doctor took down some notes as she was listening, and then asked, "How has your sleep been lately?"

Rachel was starting to feel trapped. She had not been sleeping well but had never talked about this because she felt her sleep problems were too strange to mention. In the middle of the night, the sheets of the bed and fabric of her pajamas would start to bother her. She would get out of bed and try to smooth the sheets and sometimes even change her pajamas to something else.

Rachel had no idea why so many sensations were now disturbing her. She had tried all kinds of over-the-counter sleep aids and an occasional extra glass of wine. These often worked, but she would still wake up at about two or three in the morning, tossing and turning because of the irritating feeling of the sheets and her clothing. She did not struggle with this every night, but it happened often enough that she was becoming more tired. To make up for her loss of sleep, she started to significantly increase the amount of coffee she drank to make it through the day.

When she explained this to the emergency room physician, Rachel began to realize that there was more going on in her life than she realized or even wanted to look at. The truth was that the stress of her chronic pain was starting to impact her life negatively.

The doctor asked Rachel if she displayed any other symptoms, such as an upset stomach, constipation, back pain, headaches, diarrhea, and dizziness. Rachel confessed that, yes, in fact, she had most of those symptoms off and on over the past few months. From these questions the doctor was asking, Rachel was starting to wonder if she had some other problem, maybe even cancer.

With a few more questions, the doctor gathered some general information about how Rachel felt at home with her husband and children and what type of stress she was experiencing at work. Rachel wondered if her marriage was falling apart, if she was really being the kind of mother she needed to be, and how she could keep up with the role of being a manager at work. As she talked about these three areas of her life, the feeling of that "heart attack" was starting to ramp up again.

"The problem I think you have been having," the doctor started, "has to do with stress. Over the past two years, you have had a major life change occur with your diagnosis of fibromyalgia. There are probably other stressors, but this diagnosis is a major one. Your body recognizes that you are facing challenges and is trying very hard to restore the balance that you have lost. You have probably heard of panic attacks, but do you know what the symptoms are like? They are very similar to the feeling of having a heart attack."

Rachel was shocked. Yes, she had heard of panic attacks, but she did not know why people had them. All the questions that the doctor was asking began to sink in. Since receiving the fibromyalgia diagnosis, Rachel tried very hard not to let it stop her, not to let it change her schedule or pull back from her many responsibilities, especially at home. She just pushed through the discomfort, achiness, and pain. After a few moments of silence, Rachel said, "I guess I have to rethink how I am handling my life right now. Maybe something does need to change. I feel like the heart attack symptoms are starting up again right now."

DOCTOR RECOMMENDATIONS

Rachel sat at the end of the hospital exam table in a hospital gown. She felt exposed—not just physically, but emotionally, too. She felt that the physician was telling her that she was a terrible person and that her life was a wreck. Fortunately, the doctor had great skill in delivering bad news to hurting people and was able to help Rachel see that this unexpected trip to the emergency room was an opportunity for her to recognize needs in her life that should not be ignored.

The doctor recommended that Rachel work with a psychologist specializing in chronic pain to help her understand the stress she was facing, learn strategies to manage her pain, and address the challenges she faced at work and home. Right now, Rachel could only view the stress she was under as negative, and the doctor knew this way of looking at stress needed to be changed. She also wanted Rachel to begin working with a physical and occupational therapist to guide her on what she could be doing to calm down her overly sensitive nervous system. Rachel was also encouraged to work with her primary care doctor to arrange for a few hours of medical leave from work each week so that Rachel could keep these appointments for the next several weeks while she got some of her symptoms under control.

When Rachel heard about the medical leave from work, she began to object. The doctor looked at her with a serious expression, "If you want, you can just wait until you have another panic attack. It is also possible that your next crisis will be a heart attack. How much work do you think you will miss if you have a heart attack? Rachel, your symptoms are serious, and you need to take this seriously."

Rachel was not quite ready to see what was happening to her as something she couldn't handle on her own. She wanted her life to go on as normal and still be able to get the medical help she needed. But in the end, she was willing to give it a try. "After all," she thought, "nothing else has worked, and I am only getting worse."

8

• • •

HOW ACUTE PAIN
BECOMES CHRONIC PAIN

When Rachel returned home from her emergency department visit, she was both emotionally and physically exhausted. Her husband was understandably anxious and upset; he wanted her to get a second opinion and was still convinced his wife had experienced a real heart attack. Her children were worried at first, but they soon recovered. Now that their mom was home, they wanted her to play with them and bake cookies to cheer everyone up. Rachel spent time with the kids but felt she also needed to update her other relatives. After making a few phone calls to concerned family members, Rachel curled up on the couch with a good book, read a little, and spent some time thinking. Two questions stuck out in her mind: What kind of stress was she under that led her to have a panic attack? How did she end up with chronic pain?

Within a few days, Rachel met with her primary care physician, who helped set up appointments with a psychologist, physical therapist, and occupational therapist. It was hard for Rachel to talk with her employer about getting time off, but they were more than willing to help. Rachel was a top performer, and they cared about her and the work she did. They wanted to see her healthy again.

SIGN ONE OF CHRONIC PAIN: REACTIVATION OF OLD PAIN PATHWAYS

When Rachel met with the psychologist, she needed to give a detailed history of her experiences with pain and describe the stressors in her life. These questions helped her to start thinking differently about her pain. Rachel recalled that even before she was first diagnosed with fibromyalgia two years ago, an old ankle injury seemed to come back to life. At first, she thought she must have reinjured the ankle and did not know it, but now she was not so sure.

Rachel thought back to the first time she experienced an ongoing problem with pain. She was fifteen years old, in ninth grade, and playing on the school's basketball team. Her only major injury playing basketball was a sprained ankle. But as Rachel began to think about her ankle injury, she recalled that the ankle did not heal well. She could not put weight on it for weeks and ended up missing half the season. In fact, that ankle bothered her throughout her high-school basketball career.

Now that she was learning about the role of stress in her life, Rachel had to ask herself if there was anything else going on around the time of that basketball injury. Her grades were good in school, and she had plenty of friends. Then she remembered— her brother was diagnosed with leukemia that year. Her family life came to a standstill as her parents took him to medical appointments and sought help at a large cancer treatment center several hundred miles away. Just remembering this period of her life now many years later, Rachel could still feel the weight of worry and anxiety she had both for her brother and her parents. Her brother eventually recovered, but those four years were simply a blur. There were no family vacations or fun outings. Just stress, financial hardship, and constant worry.

SIGN TWO OF CHRONIC PAIN: POOR RECOVERY FROM SURGERY

Another piece of Rachel's chronic pain puzzle appeared in her late twenties. She had been working in her chosen career since graduating from college. For her first full-time marketing position, she worked at a small marketing firm that would hire an inexperienced person like her. Eventually, she worked hard to move from small marketing firm to small marketing firm and finally to a well-known firm that worked in radio, television, and print.

She had just begun working as an assistant manager at the age of twenty-eight when she developed pain in her wrists. She was eventually diagnosed with carpal tunnel and sent for physical therapy. Looking back, Rachel recalled not taking the physical therapy seriously. She was too busy to go to the appointments or follow through on all the exercises she was supposed to do each day. She was just starting her dream job, working long hours, and she and her husband wanted to start a family. After a few physical therapy sessions, she asked her doctor if there was any other option for treatment. Not long after that appointment with her primary care doctor, Rachel was scheduled to have carpal tunnel surgery, first on her left wrist, then her right.

The surgeon gave an overview of what her recovery would look like and the steps she would need to follow. Rachel followed them faithfully, but after several weeks of recovery, she still was not healing. The pain in her wrists and hands was just as bad as it was before the surgery. When she went back to the surgeon to ask questions, he said the surgery had gone well and suggested that her problems may not be related to carpal tunnel but something else. This upset her. What other problems was he referring to? Did he know what was wrong but wasn't telling her? Why was she not healing?

It was not long after the problems with her two wrist surgeries that she began to develop numbness in her fingertips. Rachael saw a neurologist, but he did not have any clear explanation for this symptom and suggested it might be a temporary side effect from her recent surgery. He felt that when she healed completely and the upset nerves began to settle down, things would begin to turn around, and the numbness and discomfort would eventually go away.

SIGN THREE OF CHRONIC PAIN: FEAR OF PAIN

The numbness and tingling did not go away as the neurologist had suggested. Over the next few weeks, Rachel was very aware of her fingers and wrists, as well as the growing discomfort in her right ankle from her old injury. It was during this time she began to do some online research about her symptoms.

Rachel was very good at searching for information and finding what she was looking for on the internet. She came across stories of people with symptoms like hers that had undiagnosed tumors along the nerves in the spine, degenerative nerve diseases, lupus, genetic disorders, and unusual forms of cancer. The personal stories were even worse than the medical diagnoses. People had lost their jobs, marriages, and homes due to persistent pain.

Rachel began to become seriously concerned about her health and well-being. It made sense to her to do what she could on her own and see if anything helped. She tried pain creams, prescription pain patches, ointments, essential oils, and kinesiology tape. Almost everything had the same result—there were a few hours of relief, but the pain would just return to what it was before. Now she was worried that this pain was going to just be a permanent part of her life. She was afraid.

SIGN FOUR OF CHRONIC PAIN: PAIN CATASTROPHIZING

When Rachel was at work, she kept her struggle with pain to herself. She was beginning to compensate for her pain by doing her work differently, but not so differently that anyone would notice. But it was a different story when she came home from work. She arrived home exhausted, upset, and in pain. When her husband returned from work, pain was all Rachel talked about and the only thing her husband was concerned about. He, too, was worried.

Rachel discussed her pain daily with her mother on the phone and shared her struggles with her best friend. Rachel believed the support she received from her family, relatives, and close friends would be helpful in her struggle with pain. She did not realize that her choice to talk about pain actually kept pain on her mind constantly.

When Rachel thought about her pain, she would say, "This pain is killing me. It is never going to end. I am going to be just like one of those horror stories that I read about on the internet." She shared these thoughts privately with her husband. When her mother and girlfriend asked about her pain, she would tell them, in tears, how horrible her life would become if this pain problem did not get under control quickly.

SIGN FIVE OF CHRONIC PAIN: REDUCED MOVEMENT

Rachel had read on the internet that movement could irritate nerves; some of the articles she read suggested immobilizing painful areas so that the body could heal. This made sense to her, even though this was not sound or helpful advice.

She looked online for devices for her wrist and hands, learning she could get what she needed at a local pharmacy. First, Rachel tried wrist splints that she would wear in the evening and at night. Initially, the pressure of the splint seemed helpful. The first night she wore them, she actually slept better, but the real problem came during the next day. Her wrists and hands were in great pain all day—they ached and throbbed like never before. She did not want to wear the splints at work but wondered if keeping her wrists immobilized was her only option now.

She was a bit embarrassed at work to be wearing wrist splints, but she told all her workmates that it was only temporary. Due to the pain and awkwardness of working at the computer with wrist splints, she needed to change how she worked. Rachel began to use a voice recording device on her computer for writing reports and emails. She stopped taking handwritten notes during meetings, and at home, she asked her husband to take over the dirty dishes and folding the laundry. He was happy to help and felt that it was important for him to do as much for her as possible so she could recover. He felt that if she did less at home, she would recover faster, which is also what Rachel was hoping.

What Rachel and her husband did not realize was that the less she did with her wrists and hands, the more her pain would spread. Now it was not just the fingertips and wrists—the pain was spreading up both arms and sometimes causing shoulder pain. She assumed that her brain was giving her good pain management advice when it said, "Stop using your hands, wrists, and arms!" Unfortunately, the reduced movement led her to experience more pain.

SIGN SIX OF CHRONIC PAIN: PERCEPTION OF THREAT

There was no denying that pain was beginning to dominate Rachel's life. Her arms hurt from her fingertips to her shoulders. Her right leg hurt from her toes to her hip. None of it made sense. She knew something was wrong with her, but what?

Rachel widened her search for answers and became much more aware of all types of possible physical problems. She worried about her diet, her heart health, and became very aware of physical sensations like her heartbeat and how her stomach and intestines felt after a meal. Her brain was predicting pain would last for hours and days. Her mind was full of unanswered questions.

She blamed herself for letting her body fall apart and develop these aversive physical sensations. Her brain made a long list of rules—things she must do to manage pain—and an even longer list of things she should not do in order to avoid pain. Her brain had analyzed the situation and determined all the evidence suggested a strong sense of threat.

Based on the high level of threat, the brain produced a clear physical sensation of pain. "I am not okay," it told Rachel. With that, nobody had to convince Rachel that something was wrong and getting worse by the day. But Rachel did not realize that her brain might be making conclusions and recommendations based on incomplete information.

SIGN SEVEN OF CHRONIC PAIN: THE STRESS RESPONSE

Countless factors seemed to weigh on Rachel: the spreading pain, her constant worrying, her family's concern, her loss of movement, and the challenges in doing her office work and carrying out her household tasks. She was sleeping poorly and drinking more caffeine, both with multiple cups of coffee and her favorite diet soda. Unfortunately, Rachel did not know that the caffeine was increasing her pain sensitivity. The more caffeine she consumed, the more sensitive her brain became to pain, further impairing her ability to sleep well. These signs of chronic pain created a great deal of stress in her life.

As Rachel's stress levels increased, her body triggered the fight-flight-freeze response to prepare for the threats her brain warned her about. Her blood sugar levels increased, which led to her gradual weight increase. The levels of adrenaline and cortisol also increased. Her doctor had already begun to notice her increased resting heart rate and increased blood pressure. Her hands and feet became colder as her stress response rerouted her blood away from her hands and feet toward the larger muscles in the core of her body. With less blood in her extremities, her perception of pain amplified there, and her now engorged core muscles grew tense.

Rachel's immune response was the final step in triggering an ongoing cycle of chronic pain. Rachel did not have a virus or bacteria to fight off or a broken bone to repair, but her immune system became more active all the same, turning against her and attacking tissues and organs that were otherwise healthy. Rachel's immune system began to produce three troublesome effects throughout her body:

- Inflammation: Her immune system created inflammation in muscles, tissues, tendons, arteries, joints, and bones.
- Immune suppression: Cortisol began to suppress the protective functions of the immune system when defending against viruses and bacteria.
- Increased sensitivity to sensory input: The immune response began to impact the sensitivity of the five specialized sensory nerve endings designed to register changes and threats. The nerves became overly sensitive to all types of sensory input, and before long, almost anything—even a light touch—triggered pain.

These seven signs make up the cognitive, behavioral, emotional, sensory, and motor elements of the brain's neuromatrix. Once the pieces of this brain map link together to signal a serious threat, pain will be constantly produced. For Rachel to recover from her pain, all of these elements of the neuromatrix will need to be identified and modified so that a new map emerges in her brain—one that does not lead to chronic pain.

THREE SIGNS OF AN OVERLY SENSITIVE NERVOUS SYSTEM

As Rachel moved from acute pain to chronic pain, her nervous system was now set to remain in constant threat-detection mode. Rachel's central nervous system (brain and spinal cord) became overly sensitive so that almost any sensory input ranging from normal movements, such as sitting, standing, or lying down, to more subtle inputs from fabrics, breezes, or a light touching was determined to be a threat. When the brain's threat detector reacts to even the slightest sensation, the brain produces a constant pain signal and a continuous message of "I am not okay."

There are three signs that a person's pain has moved from acute pain, associated with the natural phase of healing after an injury, to chronic pain. First, the labels or descriptions associated with pain change when chronic pain takes over. Second, the person becomes sensitive to non-pain sensory input, such as input from light, sound, vibrations, gentle touch, fabric, temperature, or breezes. The third sign of an oversensitive nervous system is spreading pain. We will look at each of these three signs more closely.

SIGN ONE OF CENTRAL SENSITIZATION: CHANGING LABELS

When the nervous system is oversensitive (also called *central sensitization*) due to the immune system's impact on the nerve endings themselves, the brain will begin to get information from all the different types of threat-detection nerves at once. Instead of receiving just one type of pain signal about the painful area of the body, such as a dull ache from inflammation, the brain will produce a variety of pain signals with different sensations. What starts off as a dull ache becomes a sharp pain, which then changes to throbbing pain, becomes a burning sensation, and then maybe becomes numb and tingling. The color of the skin can change during this process as well.

When Rachel's problems with chronic pain started, she felt sore and occasionally achy. Over the past two years, this changed completely. She now has every type of pain sensation. She often started off the day sore and achy, but this turned into a burning pain that was so irritating that her skin was sensitive to the touch, and her skin in those areas would even become red.

SIGN TWO OF CENTRAL SENSITIZATION: SENSITIVITY TO NON-PAIN SENSORY STIMULATION

When Rachel began to be bothered by her sheets and pajamas, she was very confused. Looking back, she had become sensitive to more than just the sheets. When she was outside, she was much more sensitive to bright light. It seemed that she could not handle the sun at all and had to wear long sleeves and a wide-brimmed hat anytime she spent time outside. Noise from music and crowds became irritating to her and quickly caused a headache. She noticed certain fabrics caused irritation—now she wore only soft cotton fabrics. She was not able to enjoy food or drinks that were too cold or too hot. Even riding in the car or on a public bus would aggravate her pain if the roads were poorly maintained and produced vibrations.

Normally, the brain ignores the tightness of the belt around your waist, the glasses on your face, or the socks on your feet. But with chronic pain, the constant level of threat in the brain means normal sensations like these become an enemy. Here are a few of the common sensory inputs that can produce pain in chronic pain sufferers:

- Light touch
- Breezes
- Vibrations
- Sounds
- Light
- Fabric
- Types of clothing
- Sheets
- Temperature changes
- Normal movements
- Standing
- Sitting

SIGN THREE OF CENTRAL SENSITIZATION: THE LOCATION OF PAIN CHANGES

Rachel began to have pain in two areas of her body; first her ankle and then her wrists. As her pain persisted, it also began to spread. The pain in her ankle seemed to travel up her leg to her knee. Her knee ached and throbbed, and during the night it would become stiff, making her leg hard to walk on when she woke up in the morning. Then the pain moved further up her leg to her hip. At first, she assumed she was walking a bit differently due to the soreness of her knee, but then the strangest thing happened. One night, as she was going to bed in the evening, her entire right leg hurt all the way up to her hip. When she woke up, the pain had shifted to her left hip.

The changing labels of her pain sensations confused Rachel, and the increased sensitivity to normal sensory information was both surprising and upsetting. But when her pain switched sides of her body, she thought she was losing her mind. She searched her memory to figure out what might have happened in the night that caused the other side of her body to hurt.

Because of her increased sensitivity to normal sensations, Rachel purchased new sheets and special pillows advertised to help reduce pain. Then she ordered new pajamas and different underwear, hoping they would not irritate her.

On nights when she just tossed and turned in bed, she ended up on the couch in the living room. After a few nights of poor sleep in the bed and on the couch, her pain spread once again, this time across her lower back, from her right hip to her left hip. This made many everyday movements difficult. Laundry changed from being a normal hassle to a difficult, painful challenge due to all the small movements that aggravated her lower back.

Before Rachel learned about chronic pain and how her brain operates to produce pain, she did not see the problems with her lower back, ankle, wrist, hip, and leg as being linked. Like many others with chronic pain, she pursued advice and treatment from many individual medical specialists who treated each specific problem as an isolated problem. This led to many different medications and medical treatments over the years that cost both time and money. In the end, Rachel was not any healthier. The treatments mostly focused on reducing symptoms, not improving her health or helping her with the underlying problem of chronic pain.

9

· ● ● ●

THE SEVEN AMPLIFIERS OF PAIN

What David could not accept or understand was that his life as a self-made, independent, and strong man seemed to be over. It had been two years since he left work at twenty-six years old. He and his wife wanted to start a family, but instead, he was fighting workers' compensation, borrowing money from his family, and watching his wife struggle to pay the bills. All they wanted was to buy a small home and move on with life.

Instead of moving on, David focused on what he thought was helpful—getting more medical treatment. After multiple surgeries, a spinal cord stimulator, the subsequent removal of the spinal cord stimulator, physical therapy, and multiple injections, David's ability to look forward to his future, make plans, and be hopeful was gone. In any case, the pain medications he was on made it hard for him to think.

Since he could not think well and had few good things to say, he said little. When he did talk with his wife, he was irritated and unkind, even as she tried to make conversation and be encouraging. David would have benefited from talking with a rehabilitation psychologist to process all that was changing in his life, but that never happened.

Like most people, David did the best he could to manage the challenges of his life. David and his wife were both anxious and upset about their circumstances, and even more concerned about whether they could enter the next phase of their lives as new parents. But David didn't know how to talk about those topics easily.

THE ELECTRIC GUITAR

In standard medical care for pain management, practitioners focus on specific injury sites or pain syndromes, such as headaches or migraines. Less attention is paid to other factors that may influence a person's experience of pain, such as or his or her emotional state and thought processes. Instead, physical therapists focus on mechanical problems and physicians on medications, healing of tissue, and medical procedures that address a physical problem.

Even though these healthcare professionals know about the biopsychosocial approach to diagnosis and treatment, most, in actual practice, focus only on the biological factors that influence pain, ignoring psychological and social factors. The seven mindsets discussed in this chapter represent some of the key psychological and social amplifiers of pain. These often exist independent of the reactions a person may have to chronic pain. Since we have already discussed the stress response that is triggered by pain, this section focuses on many of the other life events that may be less noticeable in a person's life but still significantly impact how a person experiences pain.

If David is going to be helped with his pain, then the biological, psychological, and social aspects of his condition have to be considered together. Due to the limited focus of David's medical care on biological factors, chronic pain began to set in after the normal periods of healing and recovery from his injury and surgeries. Immediately after David's injury, it would have been important for him to learn about some of the psychological and social factors that impact healing and the experience of pain. Early interventions could have helped prevent chronic pain from developing.

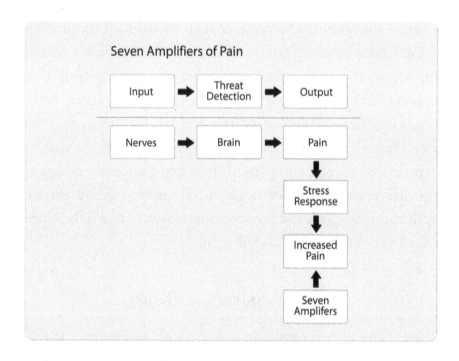

To teach patients about the psychological and social aspects of pain, I use the example of an electric guitar. An electric guitar looks similar to an acoustic guitar, but an electric guitar needs a cable connecting it to an amplifier to increase the sound of the guitar. If you lightly strum the electric guitar strings while the amplifier is turned down low, very little sound will be produced. If the amplifier is turned up high, even a very light strum of the guitar strings will produce an ear-shattering sound. It's the amplifier settings that create an intense sound or very little sound.

The electric guitar example is helpful when teaching the biopsychosocial model as it relates to chronic pain. An injury or physical problem is like the guitar. Small changes, such as inflammation, occur in the body due to some event. The inflammation is similar to lightly strumming the guitar strings.

How the brain analyzes the change caused by inflammation is influenced by many types of factors, including how a person thinks, what a person feels, and what else is happening in a person's life, such as stress. When a person's thoughts, emotions, and life situation are all negative, it is like turning up the amplifier of the guitar. Even a small physical change will be experienced as loud and painful if we experience several negative life events and have negative mindsets. Positive events, optimistic thoughts, and positive emotions turn down the amplifier so the brain produces less pain.

GATE CONTROL THEORY

There is an easy way for scientists and health professionals to talk about the pain without relying on the electric guitar metaphor—it is called the *gate control theory* of pain. Gate control theory was the first modern explanation of how pain is produced, which led to the later development of the neuromatrix model. In 1965, Ronald Melzack and Patrick Wall described two sets of nerves that influence the perception of pain.[1.] We have nerves that detect vibration, pressure, and touch, and another set of specialized nerves that detect problems and warn us of damage. If a man walks through a door and hits his shoulder hard on the door frame, the specialized nerves send a signal to the brain that something has changed. His brain will create a pain signal, letting him know his shoulder is hurt. If he rubs his shoulder, the nerves that detect vibration, pressure, and touch will send signals to the spinal cord and brain that then interfere with the other nerves sending signals that something is wrong. The rubbing action on his shoulder, therefore, will lead to a decreased sense of pain.

But rubbing a hurt shoulder is not all that reduces the experience of pain. We have an amazing chemistry cabinet in our brain that also interferes or reduces our experience of pain. Picture the spinal cord that runs up and down the back and neck as having small gates located along the sides of the spinal cord. The brain produces chemicals called endorphins when we are happy. These endorphins travel down the spinal cord into the core of our body, helping us feel good.

As the endorphins travel down the spine, they also close the gates that are along the spinal cord. When these gates close, less information about problems and damage can travel up the spinal cord back to the brain. When our level of happiness and joy is high, nerve signals that would normally lead to pain are greatly reduced, meaning the brain does not receive enough information to produce a pain signal. That is why a football player in a championship game does not recognize he is playing with a broken leg; his brain is producing too many endorphins for him to notice the damage and change signals being sent from the leg.

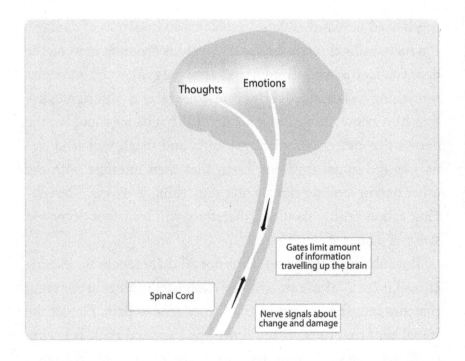

Thoughts Emotions

Gates limit amount
of information
travelling up the brain

Spinal Cord

Nerve signals about
change and damage

SEVEN AMPLIFIERS OF PAIN

There are seven mindsets involving our thoughts, emotions, and attitudes that we need to be aware of when managing chronic pain. When these mindsets are present, the gates along the spinal cord open, intensifying our experience of pain. These seven different mindsets generally have nothing to do with the injury or the condition of chronic pain itself. Instead, other life experiences, such as divorce, financial hardship, the death of someone important in your life, or a past personal history of chronic stress or trauma brings about these mindsets. The brain's neuromatrix is constantly processing information about all types of threats and challenges we face, not just information about physical pain.

MINDSET ONE: STRESS

Ever since stress has been studied by researchers, we have viewed stress as having a mainly negative impact on our mind and body. This has led psychologists and other healthcare professionals to warn the general public against the dangers associated with stress. However, this understanding of stress is only partly correct.

It is correct that stress can be damaging, especially when it is chronic or traumatic. For example, chronic and traumatic stress that occurs in childhood impacts the brain and the body's immune and hormonal systems, leading to changes in brain size, attention, concentration, memory, and emotional regulation. But there are also stressors that arise from normal life events and circumstances, such as traffic, schooling, looking for a job, new relationships, ending relationships, sickness, financial strain, and poor work environments. These stressors can be viewed in two different ways: (1) the stress is harmful to us, or (2) the stress is normal and an opportunity to grow and change. Our mindset about life stress will greatly influence the impact of stress on our health and perception of pain.

For David, a long list of stressors and a firm belief that all that he was going through was just bad luck meant fate was against him. All he could see was the bad, so he pictured his life as only getting worse. He recognized that when he thought about stress in his life, his pain increased. Unfortunately, he did not know that his mindset about stress was unhealthy or how to change it.

MINDSET TWO: ANGER

When life is unfair and we cannot reach certain goals, we can become angry. Anger can be a substitute for a wide range of other feelings that are hard to name and identify or express openly. David was angry about a number of things. He had a basic desire to see himself as a competent, capable man. He was angry at himself for making a mistake in the factory that nearly ended his life. Facing his new reality, he was also angry about his circumstances. He was sitting around the house all day, staring at the walls and trying to avoid any meaningful conversation with his wife. A life like this was unfair; this made him angry at God for having let this terrible accident happen.

David felt such intense anger that he was afraid of what he might do to himself or others. He thought it best just to keep it all pressed down and not think about it. What he did not realize was that his efforts to avoid and control unwanted feelings only intensified the emotional pressure and the physical pain he felt.

MINDSET THREE: BITTERNESS

When anger is directed toward a specific individual or life circumstance, we may spend more time wishing that others who have harmed us suffer as we have. We hang on to evidence of others' wrongdoing and wait for the day when we can present our evidence in the courtroom of life and prove the other person wrong. This process of holding on to evidence, wishing for revenge, and waiting for justice leads to constant rumination about others' wrongdoing, which is called bitterness. Bitterness is a toxic mindset that has the power to change a person's personality and increase the experience of physical pain. Often, this kind of anger is not shared with others openly, making the power of bitterness even stronger in a person's life.

David was bitter about how he lost his workers' compensation and about why he was unable to get disability assistance from the federal government. He had multiple medical visits with independent medical examiners who told him there was nothing wrong with his back and that he should go back to work. The first time he heard this, he was depressed. The second time he heard this, he wanted to kill the independent medical examiner.

Just before he was going for a review of his workers' compensation, he caught a private investigator, presumably hired by the insurance company, hiding near his home and taking pictures of him and his wife. He called the police, who did nothing to help him. He then contacted his lawyer, who told him, "This is how the game is played. Sorry." But sorry was not enough for David. He wanted to get these people back for ruining his life and accusing him of being a fraud. His mind went over these details repeatedly, especially at night when he was trying to sleep.

MINDSET FOUR: FEAR

David did not see himself as fearful. In fact, he disliked the quality of fear he saw in others and believed that he had learned to manage and overcome fear from his father, a military veteran. Despite his sense of personal strength, he still would wake up in the night, sweating, tense, and overwhelmed. He did not identify the emotion as fear, but that is what it was.

One night, as he tried to calm himself after waking up, David felt the weight of his responsibilities and his love for his wife and the family they wanted to start. He was truly afraid for his well-being and that of his family. How would they make it? What if he did not recover and his pain and medical problems only got worse? What else could he do for work if he could not use his mechanical skills and physical strength? David felt threatened but was not sure what to do or where to turn for help. His mind just kept spinning, trying to solve the problems he was facing. It did not help when David noticed his pain increased as he focused on his fear.

MINDSET FIVE: ANXIETY

Anxiety is triggered when we feel out of control. Fortunately for David, he had a number of sources of support after his injury. His parents wanted to help him, as did a number of people from work, childhood friends, and his employer. Everyone gave him the same message: "David, you are going to get through this. You can handle this. We are going to help you."

It was that message of being helped by others that bothered David the most. He wanted to be in control of his life, to be strong and independent. He did not want to be helped, not even by his parents. All the reassurance he received reminded him that he was, in fact, not in control of his life or his circumstances. As weeks turned into months, he was still recovering, and his sense of anxiety increased. He hated not having control. As with the other unwanted emotions he was currently struggling with, David relied on either avoiding the feelings altogether or controlling them. He had yet to learn that avoidance and control only increased his struggle with anxiety and made the problems worse.

MINDSET SIX: SADNESS

Sadness was not a feeling that David knew very well. He did not let himself feel sad. All David knew was that sadness just got in his way. He felt that it was best to leave the past in the past and move on.

A sign that David was, in fact, struggling with sadness was how he reacted when someone asked him if he was sad. This was especially true if his wife asked. She could read him like a book. She saw his eyes, his face, his posture, how he was breathing and knew he was sad. It seemed natural for her to ask about it. After two or three of David's explosive, angry responses to her questions about sadness, she eventually stopped asking. Like many others who find emotions difficult to handle, David replaced his sadness with irritation and anger.

David did not understand that the loss of health, mobility, and the ability to work naturally leads to sadness. With all that David was going through now, sadness was a minefield to be avoided.

MINDSET SEVEN: LONELINESS

Loneliness is painful. We are built for social connection, and not being connected with others has a negative physical and emotional impact on our health. While David appreciated the support that he was receiving, he still experienced social disconnection. He was lonely even though he was surrounded by friends and family because he felt isolated by his unusual medical condition. None of his friends had experienced a medical crisis like David's. He was tired of answering the question, "How is your pain today?" He could not explain his intense experience of pain, and he did not feel that people fully believed him anyway. This only added to his feelings of isolation and loneliness.

Rather than let himself feel his loneliness, David mostly felt angry and did not know where the anger was coming from. It was his primary care physician that noticed the changes in his mood, appetite, energy level, and sleep and suggested that David talk with one of his nurses for the last few minutes of their appointment. The doctor explained that the nurse, Sarah, had recently gone through a serious battle with cancer but was recovering well.

David was direct and irritated, "Why would I need to talk to her? Do you think I have cancer now?"

The doctor only said, "Just trust me. It might help. And no, you don't have cancer."

REFRAMING MINDSETS WITH ENCOURAGEMENT

David was uncomfortable and did not know what this nurse was going to say. She was kind and soft-spoken and asked David if she could tell him a little of what she went through in her battle with cancer. He agreed and quietly listened.

Sarah had breast cancer for two years and had both breasts removed at twenty-six, the same age David was when he was injured. She talked about the shock of having her life turned upside down, the stress affecting her family as she lost her income, and her anger about the unfairness of her condition. She described the stress her cancer caused for her two young children, the anxiety of not knowing what was going to happen next, the sadness of losing her breasts, and the fear of losing her life. And even though she had others supporting her at the time, she talked about the loneliness of fighting cancer and how she felt isolated from others who loved her.

The hard look on David's face slowly softened as she told her story. He lowered his head as tears began to form in his eyes. He felt embarrassed by emotions, but he realized that he was not alone. After a few moments of silence, David quietly said, "I am so sorry you had to go through all of that. I think I know how you feel."

"Thank you," she replied. "I know that you do."

She had given him hope that his life was not over, and like her, maybe he could find a way forward. He let the nurse give him a hug before he left the room. He found the doctor in the front office and simply said, "You were right. I needed to hear that."

STEP TWO

CALM THE NERVOUS SYSTEM

Be willing to have it so, because acceptance of what has happened is the first step in overcoming the consequences of any misfortune.

—William James (1842–1910)

With knowledge of how the brain produces pain, we can now start adjusting how the brain and body respond to pain. The techniques, strategies, and practices covered in this section are relatively simple to learn but will take considerable time to master.

The key to calming the nervous system is first recognizing when the brain and body are oversensitive and stressed. By practicing the calming strategies, you will begin to have a new awareness of what your mind and body should feel like when they are relaxed. For a person with chronic pain, it may be a new experience to have constantly tense muscles become loose and comfortable. As you begin to manage the stress that comes with chronic pain and reduce the fear associated with everyday movements, you will find that the activities which used to be associated with pain are easy to do. As your brain creates new pathways that do not link pain with activity, you will have the tools you need to start moving forward with the life you want to live.

10

• • •

TURN OFF THE THREAT DETECTOR

David's first day in the pain rehabilitation program was an emotional rollercoaster. He did not know what to think after meeting with the team members who would be taking him through the ten-week treatment program. He was so angry about his chronic pain and prior medical treatment he did not want to let a single ray of hope come into his life if it meant being disappointed again. Despite his guardedness and lack of trust, what he heard on that first visit made sense. He was greatly encouraged that healthcare professionals believed what he was going through was real. They were able to explain how chronic pain developed, which he never expected to hear. For the first time, he thought, "Maybe I am not crazy after all."

What struck him as he talked with the nurse, physician, occupational therapist, physical therapist, and psychologist was that no one seemed to be bothered by his questions, suspicion, or even his irritable mood. In fact, they validated that his concerns were right on target. They even said, "Who wouldn't be upset about developing chronic pain, losing a job, or being told the pain is in your head? Your situation is definitely not good." For reasons David could not explain, hearing their understanding response to his frustration helped him drop his guard, at least a little.

THE FLOODLIGHT AND MOTION DETECTOR

David was first informed about the pain rehabilitation program by his primary care doctor and did not recall much about what the doctor told him to expect. When David sat down with the psychologist, he was not sure why he was there at all. After all, what could a psychologist do about the pain?

David had many good qualities, including his willingness to be direct. After leading introductions and telling David how the next fifty minutes were going to proceed, the psychologist asked David if he had any questions. David's question was predictable, "No offense, but I am not sure why I need to see you. I was not expecting to meet with a psychologist. I don't have any mental health problems, as far as I know."

As with many of the other questions David had that first day, the psychologist seemed ready with an answer. David was assured that many other patients starting the program were equally surprised. But what David heard next got his interest. The psychologist asked David if his chronic pain impacted his life. Yes, of course, it did. Then she asked, "Do you think your life impacts your chronic pain?" He had never really thought about that, but immediately he realized that other things going on in his life did influence his chronic pain. He just was not sure why or how.

The psychologist asked for permission to give David an illustration that might help him see how psychology and learning about the mind–body connection might be a helpful part of his rehabilitation program. The psychologist explained the concept of an oversensitive central nervous system by describing how a floodlight and motion detector work together. Her explanation went something like this:

"David, you have probably seen a floodlight on a house, garage, or warehouse before. Many come with a motion detector that triggers the light to turn on if there is any movement in the area. When the floodlight turns on, and you see something moving through your yard, you know the motion detector is working correctly.

"However, motion detectors do not always work the way they should. For example, if a single leaf blows through the yard, and the floodlight turns on, then you have a problem with the motion detector—it is not working the way it should.

"Your central nervous system is like the motion detector. When your brain and spinal cord are working the way they should, problems are detected, and you are warned that something is not right. When your central nervous system is oversensitive, even normal activity, a light touch or sitting, can trigger pain—just like how an overly sensitive motion detector activates when a leaf falls. The problem with a malfunctioning motion detector is not the floodlight. You do not need to change the light bulbs because they keep lighting up your yard. In the same way, when your brain is oversensitive, the problem is not the pain the brain produces. The pain-detecting software in your brain is the problem.

"David, you probably injured yourself on the job before you had this severe accident. If you've ever smacked your thumb with a hammer, the nerves in your thumb and hand woke up and started sending a lot of signals to the brain. Some of this nerve activity is electrical. Picture electrical activity running through the thumb and hand and up to the brain to report on the status of your injury. This is the way your nervous system should work. As healing occurs, the electric activity in the nervous system should settle down again.

"But now imagine that the electrical activity in your hand does not settle down for some reason. Instead, the nerves keep firing rapidly, constantly sending signals and updates to the brain about everything happening in the thumb and hand, even after the tissue damage in the thumb has begun to heal. When this occurs, almost any activity will trigger the alarm system in the brain, and pain will be produced. It will be hard to hold a pen, shake a hand, put on a glove, brush your teeth, put your hand into your pocket, or have it in warm or cold water.

"If you are interested, David, the physical therapist, occupational therapist, physician, and I will help you learn how to reduce the sensitivity of your central nervous system so that normal activity, like bending or twisting, no longer leads to the experiences of intense pain you have now.

"If you were thinking that working with a psychologist was going to be like the therapy sessions you see on TV shows, well, that is not what we are going to do. I am going to give you the tools you need to manage pain better. How does that sound?"

For David, that not only was a relief—it actually sounded pretty good. David was the strong, independent type of man who viewed fear, anxiety, and depression as weaknesses. He was guarded when talking about his life and did not like the thought of needing to talk about his emotions now, especially with a stranger. But learning how to manage pain would be great. No one had explained pain in this way before—maybe there was something he could learn from the psychologist after all.

DAVID'S FIRST PRESCRIPTION

After the appointment with the psychologist, David met with the physician taking over his medical care for the next ten weeks and managing all of his medications. David was under the impression that his own physician had still not found the right combination of medications to address his chronic pain, and he was hoping this new doctor was an expert who knew just the right medications, injections, and treatments to prescribe. Just like David's meeting with the psychologist, the meeting with the physician did not go as he had expected—it went better.

The physician took a careful history of David's health, which seemed pretty routine for what doctors do. He also asked about his family background, education, work, marriage, and finances. Getting all of that information took quite a bit of time, and David could not figure out the point of all the questions. Then the doctor asked a question David was not expecting.

Looking David directly in the eye, the physician asked, "David, what would you think about getting off some of the medications you have been on?" David was in enough shock that he did not say anything for a moment. How in the world was he supposed to manage his pain without pain medication?

He finally replied, "Well, honestly, I have never thought about that. Why would I want to do that?"

The next surprise occurred when the doctor began to explain how the medications David was currently on were not working in a way that was actually helpful for the pain management

David needed. In fact, David learned that the combination of muscle relaxers, opioids, and anxiety medication he used was dangerous. He would need to be taken off most of those medications over the ten-week program, which did not sit well with David. He could feel his stress and irritation levels rising during this conversation, and he also immediately noticed an increase in his pain levels.

Meeting individually with the entire team on David's first day in the program was overwhelming. There was so much information to take in, so many ideas and concepts to absorb. Just when he thought he had heard as many strange things as he could handle, the doctor took out his prescription pad and began to write. David assumed there might be some new medication that was going to be offered. He could not have been more wrong!

As the doctor wrote, he began to talk with David about what his life would be like during the rehabilitation program. He asked David, "Do a lot of people ask you about your pain?" David explained that this was the only thing people asked him about.

Then the doctor finished writing on the prescription pad and said, "David, I've written two instructions on this prescription pad, and I want you to follow them. First, I want you to stop talking about your pain. I know that people are going to ask you about it, but when they do, just politely respond that you do not need to talk about it. Tell them you are happy to talk about other things.

"Second, I want you to avoid exaggerating when you talk about your pain, even when you talk to yourself about it. Do not say, 'This pain is killing me.' Your pain is not killing you. You would be dead by now if it was killing you.

"Do not tell people your pain is so bad you cannot get out of bed. Is pain ever so bad that you cannot get out of bed? No. Do you use a bedpan to relieve yourself because you can't get out of bed? Probably not.

"Do not say to yourself, 'This pain is an eleven on a scale of one to ten.' Your pain is not at an eleven. In fact, it probably is not even a ten. When pain is at a level ten, a person is not able to speak, is only able to scream, and is about to pass out. Your pain is probably not a ten.

"Do not exaggerate your pain—not to yourself, and not to anyone else. We have found that talking about pain and exaggerating pain keeps the brain focused on pain. We want to help you focus on getting better, and following these two instructions will help. How does that sound?"

David actually laughed out loud when he heard this prescription from the doctor. David had never said this to anyone, but he was really tired of talking, thinking, and being asked about his pain everywhere he went. For David, this prescription sounded interesting, if strange. He was not sure how his wife and parents would handle the change; they were as anxious and upset about his pain as he was. He was curious about what he would talk about if he did not talk about pain anymore. He was looking forward to finding out.

EDUCATING FAMILY MEMBERS

A problem that many pain rehabilitation patients have is explaining their treatment program to friends and family. Pain patients have people in their lives who have suffered with them through the ups and downs of treatments, surgeries, and therapies. When patients are asked to explain what treatment is like, it is often hard for them to put into words all that they have heard and are learning.

To help people communicate with family members and friends about our approach and the complicated concepts that come from neuroscience, we provide patients with simplified written information about chronic pain and the nervous system. As David heads home, we want his family and friends to become a part of the team that supports the changes that are going to be happening.

If friends and family do not understand why David is reducing his medication or doing difficult stretches and exercises, these important people in his life might work against the changes David is trying to make. Family members and friends are known for offering patients like David their own pain medications, doing all the work around the house, and getting water or snacks for them so they do not have to get up. They also are notorious for constantly talking about the pain.[1.]

This kind of help from David's family and friends needs to stop so that he can get better and follow his rehabilitation program. What family members need to offer is genuine empathy and support that helps David to have confidence, independence, and hope.[2.] To ensure this happens, David needs to ask friends and family the following:

- Please encourage me when you notice that I am doing things on my own and making progress.
- Please do not do things for me without asking me first.
- Please do not bring me food and drinks.
- Please do not do chores that I can do myself.

- Please do not tell me it is too cold, wet, windy, hot, or humid for me to take a walk outside for a few minutes every day.
- Please do not offer me medications if you see I am uncomfortable.
- Please do not ask me about my pain. Let's talk about something else.
- Please do not cancel our plans because I might have pain.
- Please do not talk to my doctor for me. I can communicate with others about what I need.
- If I start moaning, groaning, bracing myself, or sighing, please just ignore me.
- Please remind me that there is hope, look for improvements, and show kindness and support.

WHERE TO START

As you work on your own recovery and rehabilitation from pain, you will find that movements, stretching, weight-bearing exercises, walking, biking, and regaining balance and strength will increase your pain. Your automatic strategy for handling pain might be to quickly turn to the chiropractor for an adjustment, take prescribed or over-the-counter medication, use medical marijuana, or schedule trigger-point injections.

These decisions can limit your brain and body from learning how to manage pain without these aids. Even the common problem of not sleeping works in a similar manner. If a person has difficulty sleeping and automatically turns to a sleep medication from a drugstore, such as melatonin, the brain's melatonin production will shut down as the person starts to regularly use pills each night. This creates a dependence on the medication, but more importantly, it also creates the mindset that the person with sleep difficulty cannot function or learn to overcome the sleep problem on their own.

There are two key concepts of chronic pain management: (1) When we choose passive solutions, such as medications, to solve problems, we might get short-term relief, but we miss out on the opportunity to learn actionable strategies that can improve our health. (2) When we choose solutions that help reduce pain in the short term, we create additional long-term problems. Effective pain management strategies are active and help move us toward health, even if they leave us with discomfort in the short term. Pain does not equal harm. We need to work at developing a mindset that "motion is lotion"; we cannot get better without finding ways to move safely, stretch, and increase our activity. In the chapters that follow, we will look at ways to help calm an oversensitive nervous system and make movement less painful.

11

· ● ●

BALANCING THE PAIN SCALE

While waiting for a stoplight, a large pickup truck slammed Nancy's vehicle from behind, pushing her out into the intersection, where she was hit again from the right side by another vehicle. This accident took place over twenty years ago, but for Nancy, it seems like only a few weeks have passed. Since the accident occurred, life came to a standstill. After multiple attempts at treatment, she had given up.

Like other patients starting the pain rehabilitation program, Nancy had mixed feelings about attempting one more pain treatment approach. She had already been on several different migraine medications, most of which made her nauseous and unable to work. She wondered what the point of taking medication was if she could not function well enough to work and help her family. After several attempts by a neurologist to treat her migraines with medication, she went to physical therapy, which seemed to help. But her insurance limited the number of treatments she could receive, and she could not pay the out-of-pocket costs, so her physical therapy stopped.

She eventually went back to her primary care physician and was given a migraine medication she could tolerate, two different over-the-counter medications for headaches, and a muscle relaxer for her neck and shoulders. She knew that when her neck and shoulders flared up with pain, a migraine was not far away. Immediately after the accident, she only had migraines once per month. Over time, they became more frequent, happening twice a month, then once per week, and now four times a week. She eventually needed to cut back her work to part time so he could manage her pain. It did not make sense to Nancy, but when she cut back on her work hours, her headaches and migraines seemed to get worse. Like many chronic pain sufferers, she wrongly thought that by guarding herself from pain, she would have less pain.

THE PAIN BALANCE SCALE

When Nancy told her story to the pain rehabilitation team, they all had the same strange response. They each smiled and said something like, "Oh yes, that makes sense. As you do things to protect yourself from pain, your brain ends up becoming more sensitive to pain." Nancy thought to herself, "I know I understand English well, but I have no idea what they just said! Why in the world would protecting myself make my pain worse?" What Nancy had not yet learned was how her brain decides when to produce pain.

Based on Nancy's current understanding of pain, her headaches and migraines came on because something was wrong with her body. What this something was, she did not know, but she was convinced that only strong medication and being in a dark room would work to manage the pain. To reshape Nancy's understanding, the different team members began by talking with her about a balance scale in the brain that constantly weighed the credible evidence for danger against the credible evidence for safety.

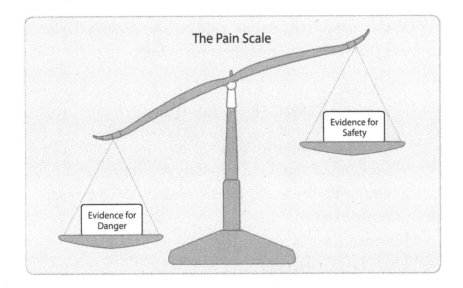

The team explained that the brain would produce pain based on which side of the scale had more weight. If there was more credible evidence of danger than there was credible evidence of safety, then the brain would produce pain. If there was more credible evidence of safety than there was credible evidence of danger, the brain would not produce pain. Nancy was intrigued. What counts as credible evidence of danger? How does "evidence" relate to her headaches? It did not make sense.

The perception of pain depends on the balance between two different types of analysis. When the brain concludes there is a good reason to believe that danger exists, the brain protects us by producing pain to warn about the danger. This way of understanding pain was best described by Lorimer Moseley and David Butler: "We will experience pain when our credible evidence of danger related to our body is greater than our credible evidence of safety related to the body. Equally, we won't have pain when our credible evidence of safety is greater than our credible evidence of danger."[1.] Moseley suggested these typical statements from chronic pain patients provide the brain evidence that there is a problem worth noting:

DANGER-IN-ME (DIM)

- My MRI is abnormal.
- The doctor said this is the worst case she had ever seen.
- Strong medication hardly helps my pain, which means my problem is serious.
- If I move, it hurts.
- I have a scary diagnosis.
- My mother had the same problem.
- I am not okay and do not feel okay.
- I need a walker or a cane to function.
- Only a "magic bullet" cure will help.

Each of these pieces of evidence points to a problem. When the brain gets enough evidence that there is a problem, it only has one reasonable choice—protect the person by producing pain to limit activity and avoid further damage.

An important question needs to be asked about DIM evidence: Is the brain making a conclusion that there is really a threat based on complete and accurate information? One of the main strategies of effective pain management is providing the brain with more accurate information about what is happening so that the brain is not constantly producing a threat response.

Safety-in-me messages are necessary for the brain to balance the scales toward hope. When hope becomes a part of a person's thinking and beliefs, the problems they have with chronic pain begin to look different. Following are some of the many safety-in-me messages that help create hope:

SAFETY-IN-ME (SIM)

- Pain does not equal harm.
- I can be sore but safe.
- Motion is lotion.
- Pacing is progress.
- I can break the brain's protective rules and still be okay.
- I am okay, and I am getting better.
- My back is strong.
- I can be active even with pain.
- I can rewire my brain.
- Medications and surgeries are not effective for everyone.
- Medical testing (MRI, CT scans, x-rays) does not tell the whole story.

SIM messages cannot just be repeated by a person with chronic pain to magically reduce pain. We are convinced of something by experiencing the new reality directly. This is why movement, exercise, stretching, strength conditioning, and developing new movement habits play such a critical role in bringing about change in a pain rehabilitation program. We do not really know that "motion is lotion" or that "pain does not equal harm" until a person who has been sitting in bed for years begins to use an exercise bike, treadmill, elliptical, or pool—or simply starts to walk around the house—and experiences the truth. Movement soothes the joints, bones, muscles, and ligaments of the body. Pain that comes with this new movement does not mean damage is being done. There is no harm being done with most pain. Movement is necessary for our emotional and physical well-being. We can never feel well, be strong, or have our nervous system operate correctly without movement.

NANCY'S DIM MESSAGES

When Nancy sat down with the psychologist, the psychologist got out a large notepad and wrote "danger-in-me" at the top of the page. He then said to Nancy, "I am not sure if you recognize some of the danger-in-me messages that you have about your pain, but I am going to start listing some of the specific statements that you have made in our recent sessions and in today's session." The psychologist wrote down the following statements Nancy had recently made:

- Headaches and migraines run in my family.
- I have MRIs that show the damage in my neck, and the images look bad.
- I have seen the best neurologists, and they cannot help me.
- Powerful medication is needed to manage my pain, which means my problem is serious.
- Nothing helps my pain, which means my problem is serious.
- My brother is a physician, and he told me that medication is the only way to manage my pain.
- Pain stops everything I do.

- I had to get treatment in the hospital and emergency room, which is serious.
- I will never be able to enjoy dancing again.
- Pain is making me lose my friends and reduce my work.

After he completed the list and showed it to Nancy, she sat quietly for a few minutes. She finally spoke, and said, "I have made every one of those statements. I do not like the look of that list at all. I was about to argue with you that I am right to believe each of these, but as I looked at this list, I started to develop a headache, the kind that ramps up to being a migraine. That is when it hit me—just looking at this list is tipping the balance of the pain scale in my brain! If I focus on these statements and believe them, I am going to end up back in the emergency room!"

With this insight, Nancy had a slight shift in her thinking, but she wanted to ask about some of the evidence on the DIM list that seemed very convincing to her. She started off saying that the MRI of her neck was a "medical fact." It showed her where the pain in her neck was coming from. She then talked about the doctors she had seen, the neurologist who specialized in migraines. If these special doctors could not help her, didn't that mean she was beyond help and that her pain is truly chronic? What about her brother? He, too, was a physician and someone she trusted; he warned her that going off her medication would make things worse.

The psychologist reminded her that she did not have to be persuaded or convinced of anything. But he did ask her two sets of questions: (1) Did she think that her current set of beliefs was helpful? (2) What would happen if her experience in the pain program gave her a different set of beliefs about pain? Would that be okay?

She thought for a moment and confessed that her current beliefs were probably not helpful at all. The DIM messages she had in mind kept her anxious, fearful, and dreading a future of chronic pain. She also thought that letting experience help her develop new beliefs sounded better than trying to argue about the beliefs she currently had.

EDUCATION ABOUT MEDICAL TESTS

Having presented pain education to many people in the past, the psychologist knew that the education he provided was sometimes well received, with the patient having an open mind about learning new information. He also knew that some people are not convinced that their medical testing should not be the only evidence used to explain chronic pain. In fact, some people even became upset at anyone trying to suggest anything different. Regardless of the possible reactions to the topic, he wanted people to be informed so they could weigh the evidence they received from healthcare professionals more carefully and thoughtfully.

He started by explaining the questionable reliability of interpreting medical testing. A recent study was conducted where the MRI results of a sixty-three-year-old woman with lower back pain were sent to ten different MRI centers that have physicians interpret the findings.[2.] The researchers knew exactly the type of back problem the woman had when the MRI was taken: She had a disc herniation, spondylolisthesis, and severe spinal stenosis.

Based on the results from the ten MRI centers, it was clear that many of the findings that were reported were not even close to the woman's actual lower back problems. The ten MRI centers reported forty-nine different diagnoses, 45 percent missed the spinal stenosis, 47.5 percent missed the disc herniation, and 72.5 percent missed the nerve root compression. Unfortunately, most patients and many physicians do not know that the MRI is not recommended by the American College of Physicians and the American Pain Society to manage lower back pain. According to these experts, the MRI is not reliable enough to use to diagnose back problems.[3.]

Another piece of the medical testing puzzle is the fact that many people, regardless of their age and whether or not they have pain, have abnormal MRIs. Due to the normal process of aging, our spine will compress over time, which explains why we get shorter as we age. The compression occurs because our discs are deteriorating. Even though our discs are deteriorating, and we all develop arthritis in our larger joints as we age,

Degenerative Disc Disease

Age (Years)	20	30	40	50	60	70
Disc Degeneration MRI Findings	37%	52%	68%	80%	88%	93%

(See reference 4. in Endnotes)

most people do not experience pain related to the normal aging process.

With every decade, there is an increased number of people who show signs of disc degeneration.[4] You might think this also means that we have increased reports of pain with every decade, but we do not. The people who report the most pain are those in their forties. People in their sixties and seventies have far more problems with disc degeneration and arthritis, but as people age, they actually report less pain and seek help for pain less often than those who are younger. Those in their forties, followed by people in their fifties, experience more pain and seek treatment for it more often than any other age group.

The difficulty with medical testing is the impression it makes on a patient. Most people in their forties and fifties have disc degeneration and arthritis, and most of these people function well and are not limited by pain or back problems. Imagine a person in this age group is helping a friend move from one house to another, and in the process, he strains his back. He goes home, takes ibuprofen, puts ice on his back, and then tries to avoid irritating it further.

A week later, he goes to the doctor for persistent back pain, and the doctor orders an x-ray or MRI. The results come back, and the doctor says, "Looks you have some disc degeneration and signs of arthritis. That might explain the persistent pain." Soft tissue damage from moving heavy objects could also explain the pain, but that was not mentioned. All of a sudden, this man with back pain becomes a man with a bad back. Now that he as a "bad back," he changes his habits to protect his back in all activities. He begins to worry about hurting himself. He starts to walk differently and becomes anxious about any sensation coming from his back. Over time, his back becomes deconditioned, which is a nice word for being out of shape.

Many pain patients who have not had surgery view surgery as their best chance at a pain-free life. Surgery is viewed as a magic bullet. But patients who have had surgery for pain know that the results can be anything but certain and can create additional, unexpected problems. There is now plenty of research evidence that shows surgery for different types of common problems (back, neck, and knee pain) does not produce a guaranteed pain-free future. Studies have shown that the use of surgery, narcotics, and injections for back pain has comparable results in providing patients with a sugar pill (a placebo).[5.]

When people are injured on the job, at least 66 percent will return to work if they do not get surgery, but only 27 percent return to work if they decide to get surgery.[6.] Another study looked at knee surgeries. When comparing four different types of knee surgery with a completely fake surgery, there was no difference between the actual surgeries and the fake surgeries in regards to pain relief or the amount of improvement in functioning.[7.] A fake or sham surgery is a surgery where the doctor opens up the knee as if a real surgery is going to take place, but nothing is done. The patient, who is a part of a research study, is not told if the surgery was real or fake. Even with fake surgeries, patients report improved function and less pain.

PROMOTING SIM MESSAGES

As Nancy gained knowledge about pain and put into practice new routines of daily exercise, stretching, strength training, and a variety of breathing and mindfulness exercises, she began to see small changes in her headache and migraine patterns. The headaches no longer lasted twenty-four hours a day, and the migraines occurred once or twice a week, rather than four times a week. As she began to sleep better, she reported to her pain rehabilitation team, "I do not know what is happening, but something is changing. People who have not seen me in a while are saying that I look better. I really do not know what they see is different, but I do feel that something is different." But even with this progress, Nancy was still not sure it would last. Plus, there was still the pain she felt on a daily basis.

Nancy's psychologist encouraged her to recognize that the thoughts running through her mind about the future should be challenged. As Nancy pictures her day, her brain creates a variety of rules for her to follow. The psychologist explained, "Nancy, you often feel that you cannot go out of the house because your pain is going to get worse. Your brain tells you that if you go out, you are going to have more pain and that you better take your prescribed medication early in the day because the pain is going to last all day."

The psychologist suggested that Nancy's brain was not simply trying to protect her. It was rehearsing what she will do and how things will go. He said, "Before a live performance of a play, the acting cast rehearses everything that will happen on the stage. That is exactly what your brain is doing—it is rehearsing how your day will go, which your brain predicts will be bad."

This struck Nancy hard. She realized that her brain has been rehearsing a painful story for her to follow for the past twenty years. It was hard for her to imagine her day unfolding any differently than it always had unfolded. As she thought about her brain's "rehearsal," she decided to change one small element of her very familiar story.

PASSING THE TEST

The next morning, when she started her day working part-time and running errands, she decided that she was going to leave all her headache medication at home. The moment she made this decision, she could tell that her brain was warning her, "Don't break the rules! You know what could happen if you don't have your medication nearby. What if you are out running errands and you end up in so much pain you can't get home? Wouldn't that be terrible?" Nancy had been practicing the habit of thanking her mind for its kind and helpful input, but then she calmly went about her day without carrying her medication.

At the end of her first day of not carrying medication, Nancy had to admit that she was nervous several times throughout the day, but she made it. Nothing terrible happened. This small victory opened the door for one more shift in her thinking—one that would turn out to be life-changing.

The first Sunday night of December, Nancy went to bed, falling asleep quickly and deeply. Around 2:00 a.m., she woke up with a headache. This was not good. She fell back to sleep and woke up at 4:00 a.m. with the beginning of what seemed to be a migraine. She used her breathing exercises, got out of bed and stretched, and was actually able to fall back to sleep. At six o'clock, she was wide awake with her typical migraine. She could hear her brain make the prediction that the pain would last all day, that she needed her medication, and that it would be best if she just canceled her plans so she could focus on staying at home and lying down in a dark room.

Nancy got out of bed, dressed, and started her day wondering what she was going to do. She had a full day of getting her house ready for guests, shopping, and visiting a friend planned. After debating in her mind about what to do, she decided to go about her day and get everything done. If she ended up getting sick, throwing up, or feeling unable to function, she would just have to deal with it when it happened. Instead of packing her medication in her purse, she put in a paper bag for throwing up.

As Nancy recounted the story to the psychologist on her next visit, she said, "I am not sure when the migraine passed. I was so focused on getting things done that somewhere around noon, I realized the migraine was gone. I did not feel great, but I could function well enough, and I just kept going. I did my exercises in the afternoon, walked in the evening, but never needed to take medication." As Nancy was sharing this exciting event with the psychologist, he wrote down for her the new set of beliefs she had developed about safety:

- Rules can be broken.
- Motion is lotion.
- Pain does not need to stop me.
- I will be okay when I start to have pain.
- MRIs are not proof of pain and disability.
- Time with friends and family is important.
- Self-care is health care.
- There is no substitute for regular exercise.
- Pacing is progress.

The psychologist illustrated for Nancy once more the danger and safety scale. After quite a bit of work, Nancy had collected enough evidence for safety that the scale was now balanced in a new direction. She now had more evidence for safety than for danger.

As Nancy looked at her list of SIM messages and the image of the scale, she realized that what she believed about her pain at the beginning of the pain program was no longer correct. All the talk, written information, and explanations were interesting, but they did not persuade her that her life could be different. It was her own experience of seeing the reduction in stress that came with the hard work of exercise, stretching, breathing, and strength training that gave her evidence she needed to take a risk and make changes.

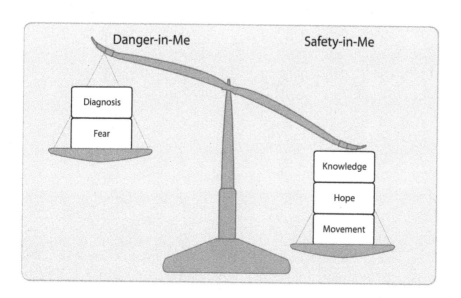

12

•••

PROGRESS THROUGH PACING

David, who was introduced in the first chapter, was twenty-six years old when a disc ruptured in his lower back while at work. Before starting pain rehabilitation, he had two surgeries to repair his back, surgeries to implant, replace, and remove an electronic stimulation device for his spine, steroid injections, and physical therapy. Some of these interventions brought short-term relief, but nothing helped improve his functioning. David kept pursuing any treatment that was recommended—he was a man of action, a doer. He had one goal in mind: find a way to get better.

It was clear that before David's injury he was a physically strong man. His handshake was crushing, and his shoulders were broad and strong. It was easy to picture him pulling a 1,000-pound load with a hydraulic floor jack across a factory floor. He did not have any difficulty walking immediately after his injury pulling the floor jack, just localized lower back pain. Back then, he was hopeful surgery to repair his ruptured disc would set everything right in his back and he would soon return to work.

After his first surgery, he woke up to pain shooting down his right leg. He was told the pain would go away as he healed in the next few weeks, but it did not. He made an appointment with the surgeon, hoping to get an explanation. He was shocked by the conversation about his post-surgical pain. The surgeon dismissed his pain as a serious concern and angrily said, "I have repaired your ruptured disc. The surgery went well, and there is nothing wrong with your back. It takes time to heal, and you are just not being patient. I cannot help that. There is nothing more I can do for you." David was too stunned to respond and later was actually glad that he did not say what he was really thinking. When David realized that the surgeon no longer wanted anything to do with him, his anger began to boil.

SETTING EXPECTATIONS

David used a cane when he arrived at my office. He had difficulty walking, standing up straight, or sitting for any length of time. David, while not happy about his chronic pain, was clearly motivated to do the rehabilitation work needed to get better. It would be fair to say he was desperate to recover. In the time that he was at home recovering, he managed to slowly remodel a bathroom, replace some windows, and change the landscaping around the house. If David had a good day with a little less pain, his to-do list was always ready and waiting for him. The only problem was that after one day of light work, he was out of commission and in bed with ice packs on his lower back and right leg to calm down the pain, redness, and inflammation that always followed.

As David's physical and occupational therapists asked questions and developed a picture of what David's life was like at home, they put together a treatment plan that would address the injured areas of his back, nerve problems associated with his injury and surgeries, and correct the habits he had developed over the past two years of compensating for his pain. Using a cane, a back brace, leaning forward, sleeping in a reclining chair, and limping all were making his pain worse, not better.

During the physical and occupational therapy assessment, the therapists asked David about his goals for the program. He stated that he wanted to be back to work in the next two months. His long-term disability was coming to an end, and he had no plans to go on permanent disability and no interest in taking narcotic drugs to manage his pain. He wanted to see results and was going to do the work necessary to make that happen.

While his focus on getting better sounded good, both of his therapists knew that getting back to work in two months might not be realistic. David was obviously a driven individual with expectations, which meant he was going to be a challenge. All the work that he had accomplished at home pointed to the possibility that David pushed himself too hard in order to accomplish what he wanted, despite having a great deal of pain. This pattern of pushing hard only made his recovery and pain levels worse. David, on the other hand, thought that pushing through pain to get work done would help him get better faster. He did not realize that his hard work prevented him from healing well and resulted in more pain interventions that caused additional problems of their own.

GOING SLOW GETS THERE FASTER

To help David, the physical therapist decided to spend extra time educating him about his nervous system. She would introduce him to the concept of *pacing*—limiting time spent on the activity and introducing periods of rest and recovery before resuming the activity again.[1.] In order to get David's buy-in, she needed to make sure he understood that the fastest route to getting what he wanted meant going slow.

Prior to David's injury and the onset of chronic pain, he was able to engage in activities for many hours over several days before he ever felt discomfort or pain. The physical therapist asked David how long he was able to work without feeling pain before he was injured. He replied that he often worked ten- to twelve-hour shifts, doing heavy physical work the entire time. He could remember being sore some nights but would never have a great deal of pain.

On a blank piece of paper, the physical therapist drew a picture of a tall mountain with a stick figure, David, climbing up the side of the mountain. She then drew two lines at the top of the mountain. The lower line represented David's discomfort threshold, and the upper line, one inch above, represented his pain threshold. She pointed to the stick figure on the side and said, "David, this is you on the side of the mountain. In the good old days before your injury, you could work for hours every day and hardly get close to the discomfort threshold. You enjoyed work, soreness did not bother you, and you were physically strong."

The therapist then drew another mountain peak to the right of the first mountain. The mountain peak was just as high, but she drew the discomfort threshold down near the base of the mountain and pain threshold just an inch up from the discomfort line. She then explained that after an injury or the onset of chronic pain, the discomfort threshold and pain threshold are both much lower and will be reached in a matter of minutes, not hours. David completely agreed. He could hardly walk or stand for ten minutes without a lot of discomfort. If he pushed through and tried to ignore the discomfort, his pain flared up quickly. Looking at these two lines at the base of the mountain, David felt discouraged. How was he going to recover when he kept being trapped by pain?

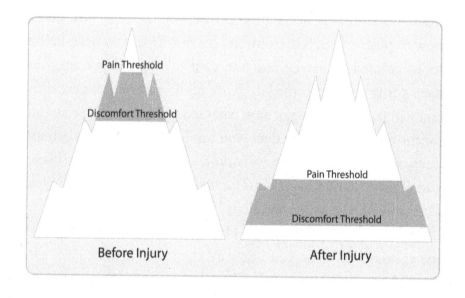

PAIN FLARE-UPS

The physical therapist asked David if she had permission to guess about how David approached his day and explore why his pain flared up. David was curious and agreed. She smiled and said, "Let's see. You don't sleep well most nights, and you use a recliner for a bed. Occasionally, a better night of sleep comes along, and you wake up, have a good breakfast, and actually feel like a normal human being again. Then you remember—you have a long list of things on your to-do list. Since you are feeling good, and the sun is shining outside, you get started on your list. You tell yourself that you are not going to do anything too strenuous, and you don't. A paintbrush is not heavy. A rake is not heavy. You are not lifting anything heavy or pulling 1,000 pounds, so you're sure you can do this easy stuff.

"You work all morning till noon, eat lunch, and go back at it. Then, around three or four in the afternoon, you are in a lot of discomfort. This is not a problem for you, because you know how to push through discomfort. By this time, you have half a room painted or maybe half the yard raked, and you need to keep going and finish the job. Around dinnertime, you are officially in pain. You are not sure what led to the sudden pain, but for the next two or three days, you can hardly move. You cannot sleep, it is hard for you to walk, and you become both irritable and depressed, making it hard for your family to be around you. Does any of that sound familiar?"

"Wow!" David exclaimed. "Have you been taking a video of me at home? How do you know all this? This is what I do. On good days, I push through. Then I pay for it. But you can't expect me to just sit around! That is why I get depressed. I have to work."

The therapist then drew a steep line that went from the discomfort threshold up to the pain threshold and then back down again. "This line," she explained, "represents your pattern of feeling good, pushing through discomfort, and needing to stop all activity for several days in order to recover. You make a little progress up the mountain when you push yourself, but then you're back at the bottom. What if I told you there was a better way?"

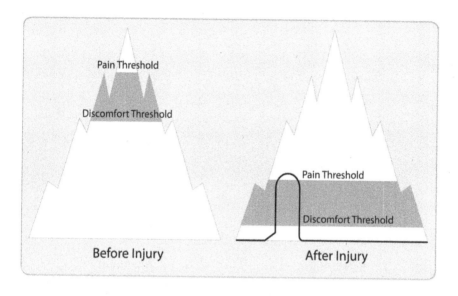

PRINCIPLES OF PACING

The physical therapist did a good job of making David curious. How did she know that this was his life? What was he supposed to do differently? She explained that what was missing from David's approach was pacing—limiting the time spent in an activity and introducing periods of rest and recovery before resuming the activity again. The therapist pointed at the discomfort threshold line on the mountain representing his life with chronic pain. She explained that pacing involves limiting the amount of time spent in the discomfort zone to a set amount of time, such as ten minutes, and then resting for another set amount of time, such as fifteen minutes. The length of time spent in an activity should be about 50 percent of a person's maximum ability to perform an activity. If a person can only walk for ten minutes with limited pain, then the target for pacing should be five minutes of walking followed by rest and recovery.

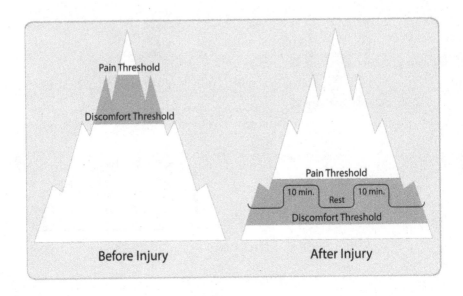

If David were to begin to follow this new pacing pattern, two important changes would take place. First, David's brain would be able to experience small amounts of normal activity, and his brain would not associate that activity with pain, only a limited amount of discomfort. This might not seem significant, but David's brain will need plenty of new experiences to loosen the connection between movement (activity) and pain. Right now, if David even thinks about walking for fifteen minutes, his back and legs hurt. He needs to break the connection between movement and pain. The only way to break the connection is by limiting his activity to short periods of time so he can move with only limited discomfort. As the connection between pain and movement loosens, David's brain will learn the important message, "Pain does not equal harm."

The second change that will occur when David starts to implement pacing is his discomfort and pain thresholds will gradually start to increase. On the image of the mountain, the lines will start going back up toward their original position.

Time spent pacing will eventually begin to shift the perception of pain in David's brain. Rather than walking for just five minutes with a limited amount of discomfort, he will soon be walking ten minutes without any additional discomfort. In the meantime, he will also be getting stronger, developing better cardiovascular health, getting more oxygen to his brain and body, and increasing his stability. All this should happen without too many pain flare-ups.

The therapist emphasized that by following the principles of pacing, David would be able to adjust upward both his discomfort and pain thresholds, but only if he goes slowly and rests. Just going slowly or only resting won't be enough. Going slowly,

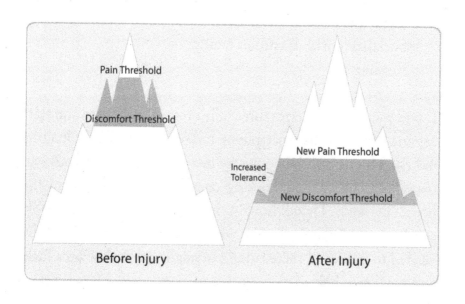

resting a short period of time, and getting back to the activity again will be needed for progress to be made.

THE PRACTICE OF PACING

Pacing can be applied to a wide variety of daily activities. The following are some household and work activities that can be the focus of pacing:

- Laundry
- Computer work
- Dishes
- Vacuuming
- Driving a vehicle
- Walking
- Exercise
- Time spent on a hobby
- Yardwork
- Time spent sitting at a desk
- Socializing with friends or family
- Reading

David was asked to select three of his regular activities and start using a timer on his smartphone to keep track of how long he did the activity and how long he rested. David chose walking, household chores, and working on repair projects around the house. Privately, David thought the idea of pacing was probably good for some people, but he was not convinced that he really needed to follow all these rules. He might try to slow up a little and see if that helped.

The therapist asked David if he thought he would have any trouble following through with the pacing exercise. Yes, he admitted. The therapist gave David the printed instructions and illustrations on pacing and asked David to bring his wife into the next physical therapy session so she could learn the principles as well. The physical therapist knew that when family members are given education about the rehabilitation process, they could be helpful at home with encouragement and reminders.

On the first day of using the pacing principles, David set the timer on his smartphone for five minutes and started vacuuming. It seemed like only a few seconds went by and the alarm went off. Time to rest. He turned off the vacuum and wondered what he was supposed to do now. Then he remembered the instructions: resting does not have to be sitting around doing nothing—although it can be that. He decided to have some coffee and read up on the news. Ten minutes later, he was back to vacuuming for another five minutes. When the alarm went off a second time, he was convinced this pacing principle was not going to work. He felt like a horse being held back by a set of reins, unable to run. Yet, he pressed on with the program. It took him three times as long to vacuum the family room and living room, which annoyed him. He felt silly resting, especially when he did not have pain.

With a few days of practice at pacing and encouragement from his wife, David crossed over the line of doubt and frustration and started to see the benefits of pacing. The most noticeable change was that his sleep improved. Because David was less flared up during the day, he began to feel better in the evening, falling asleep faster and sleeping longer. He could not believe the change.

His wife also changed. She became more relaxed and happier because David was easier to talk to and be around in the evenings. David had not realized how his chronic pain, irritability, and depression had impacted others. He was now even more motivated to go slow, rest and recover, and go slow again. "Pace it, don't race it" became his new moto.

Over the next few weeks, David increased the length of time he could spend on activities and significantly increased his tolerance for discomfort and pain. He was proud of the effort he put into his recovery, and more importantly, he began to sense there was hope that he would be able to return to work. He might not be able to move in the same way he did in the past, but he believed he could still make a contribution and enjoy being productive again at his worksite.

13

• • •

APPLY THE BRAKES ON STRESS

Rachel's life was busy, to say the least. Parenting, marriage, career, health, hobbies, and relationships were all ranked as top priorities in Rachel's mind. She was a driven perfectionist and loved to see results. But as we saw earlier, Rachel's approach to life also came at a cost. That is why she ended up in the emergency room with heart attack symptoms during a panic attack. She also struggled with her diagnosis of fibromyalgia, but the panic attack was one added problem too many. What was happening to her? Was she falling apart and not going to make it? This scared her, which might be just what she needed to slow down and examine her life.

It is not easy for pain sufferers to start a pain rehabilitation program. People with chronic pain are not only blamed by others for their problems, but they also blame themselves. Rachel was doing a pretty good job of blaming herself for her fibromyalgia and recent panic attack when she arrived for her psychology appointments in the pain rehabilitation program. Her mind was full of self-blaming thoughts: "I should have done this," "I should have done that," and "If only I had done more." As she sat down with the psychologist, all the noise in Rachel's head made it hard for her to follow the conversation with the psychologist.

DIRECTING ATTENTION

After the initial two sessions focused on pain education, the psychologist asked a relatively simple question as they started their session together. He asked, "Do you have any difficulty focusing your attention?" Rachel wanted to give the nice-sounding answer, "No, not at all!" It was important to Rachel to look good. Instead, she honestly replied, "I just don't know anymore. It is hard for me to focus my attention. I read an article and get halfway through it, and I am not sure what I am reading and have to start all over. I feel like my mind is in a fog most of the time. It was never like this before—I don't know what happened to me."

The psychologist briefly described fibro-fog, a common symptom of fibromyalgia that includes misplacing objects, difficulty following conversations, forgetting plans, and being easily distracted. The most likely causes of fibro-fog are poor sleep and lack of oxygen in the brain. To help Rachel, the psychologist introduced an exercise that would improve her attention and management of stress.

THE STRESS RESPONSE

To introduce the stress management and attention-strengthening exercise, the psychologist started with a basic review of the body's stress response. He explained that when we are under stress, our breathing rate goes up from twelve breaths per minute to twenty or more breaths per minute. This happens automatically. Even though breathing is automatically controlled by the brain, how fast we breathe is not. We can consciously slow down our breathing rate.

When we begin to slow down the breathing rate, we activate the parasympathetic nervous system and put the brakes on the stress response. The slow breathing signals the sympathetic division to take the pressure off the gas pedal of the entire stress response. When the pressure is off the gas pedal, the heart rate begins to slow down, blood pressure decreases, blood circulation returns to the hands, stomach and intestine functioning begins to return to normal, and tension decreases throughout the body.

DIAPHRAGMATIC BREATHING

The diaphragm is a large muscle at the base of the lungs that separates the lungs from the stomach cavity. As we breathe using the diaphragm muscle, the muscle will push down and draw the base of the lungs toward the stomach, creating a vacuum for air to rush into the lungs. The sign that you are using the diaphragm muscle is that your stomach will move outward as you breathe in. For babies, this is a natural way of breathing, but we adults seem to have developed the poor habit of using our ribs, chest, and shoulders to draw in the air we need. Using the chest and shoulder muscles creates tension in the upper body and can even press on sensitive nerves in the neck and shoulder region, leading to muscle tightness and pain.

Breathing with the diaphragm will allow you to get the maximum amount of oxygen in a relaxing manner. This method of breathing is often practiced by actors, singers, radio and TV personalities, and public speakers. It is very effective for helping people in stressful situations to stay calm and get the oxygen they need to perform well. It also helps people with chronic pain to turn off their stress response.

STEPS FOR DIAPHRAGMATIC BREATHING

1. Practice breathing in slowly through your nose while your hand is placed on your stomach. As you breathe in, picture the bottoms of your lungs moving down toward your hips. You might also try picturing the air filling up a balloon in your stomach.

2. As you are breathing in, put some pressure on your stomach with your hand and have your stomach push back as the air is coming into your lungs. Your stomach should move outward as you breathe in, and you should see your hand move out as the stomach moves. If your hand is not moving, put your other hand on your chest. If the hand on your chest is moving as you breathe in, then you are not using the diaphragm quite yet. With practice, you will eventually feel the stomach move outward. It can be helpful to lay on your back on a flat surface, put a large, heavy book on your stomach, and practice letting your stomach push the book up and down as you breathe.

3. To practice breathing out, you will need to purse your lips and slowly blow the air out of your lungs. Try to picture a lit candle out in front of you at arm's length. As you breathe out, imagine that your breath makes the flame of the candle

flicker just a little bit. It is not a strong exhalation of the breath, but not soft and silent either.

4. The breathing cycle has three parts: (1) inhale for four counts, (2) hold the breath briefly for two counts, and (3) exhale slowly for six counts.

5. The breath in (inhalation) needs to be slow but not too deep. If you take in too much air as you breathe in, you will end up feeling dizzy and light-headed. Measure your breath in by counting to four slowly.

6. Pause for two counts while holding your breath.

7. Breathe out slowly while you purse your lips, resulting in an audible exhalation sound.

8. Practice putting all three pieces together by counting one, two, three, four in your mind, for the breath in. Then count one and two as you hold the breath. Then count one, two, three, four, five, six as you exhale.

9. Each inhale and exhale cycle using this pattern will take about ten seconds, which means you will be breathing about six times per minute.

10. Once you have the basic steps down, practice for five minutes at a time by sitting in a comfortable chair in a quiet place. You want to have as few distractions as possible so that you can fully focus your attention on your breath.

11. As you become comfortable with all the parts of this breathing pattern, you will gradually stop thinking directly about what you are doing. Then you can start directing your attention to your midsection, the part of your lower ribs and upper stomach that is moving in and out. During those five minutes, hold your attention on your midsection, noticing

only the movement of your stomach as you breathe, blocking out all other sensations or distractions.

12. While focusing on your breath, your attention will wander, which is completely normal. Every time your attention wanders, and you bring it back to focus on your breath, you strengthen your attention. Strengthening your attention is similar to strengthening your bicep muscle—a weight is lifted up, and the bicep muscle contracts. Then the weight is let down, and the bicep muscle relaxes. Every time you bring your attention back after it wanders or relaxes is like a muscle contracting. You strengthen your ability to focus your attention.

BREATHING POWER

The steps for breathing are relatively simple. Practicing does not take much time. Besides using a timer or maybe an app on your phone, there is no financial cost involved. Because breathing is so simple, it is easy to disregard it as an effective, powerful tool for stress and pain management.

Diaphragmatic breathing is free, simple to practice, and has many benefits. As a person consistently practices diaphragmatic breathing, his or her blood pressure may also lower. Some patients who practice breathing for several weeks have reduced or been taken off their blood pressure medication. Other patients report decreased neck and shoulder pain, in part because they have stopped using the chest and shoulder muscles to breathe. Diaphragmatic breathing reduces tension because proper body mechanics are used to breathe, and oxygen content is increased throughout the body. Patients also sleep better, especially as they practice in the evening before bed or use the procedure at night when they wake up and struggle to fall back to sleep.

TURNING OFF THE STRESS RESPONSE

The three main benefits of regular diaphragmatic breathing are a tuned-down stress response, changes in brain wave activity, and reduced heart rate variability. When we slow down our breathing, the brake pedal is applied to the stress response, which is so important because stress response is a major contributor to increased pain and the development of chronic pain. As we manage our stress response, we reduce inflammation and muscle tension, and restore the proper function of the immune system so that it is not turning against us.

CHANGE BRAIN WAVE ACTIVITY

One often overlooked benefit of breathing exercises is the impact on brain wave activity. We have electrical signals that help regulate brain activity. As we talk, walk, and think, our brain waves are fast, but as we focus our attention with our mind, those brain waves slow down. Listening quietly to calm music will lead to slower brain waves. When we aim our attention at a specific target and sustain our attention over longer periods of time, our brain waves become harmonious and slow. This is exactly what happens as we repeatedly practice a breathing exercise with focused attention on the breath. The longer we practice (ten to fifteen minutes at a time) and consistently practice day after day, brain wave patterns change and become more calming.

We want our brain waves to change because it alters how the brain responds to sensory information it gets from the body. In short, the brain is less reactive to negative sensory information when it is calm (has slower brain waves). Imagine you have lower back pain. Sensory information from the back will go up to the brain, and the brain will say, "Yes, we are aware of the problem in the lower back, but we are not going to react strongly to this and set off the threat-and-pain-protection system." When calm brain waves are in charge of brain activity, less pain is produced as an output.[1.]

When your brain activity is busy and uncoordinated, it is like a family heading out the door for vacation. The family is tense—everyone is trying to remember what needs to be packed—and all of a sudden, someone bumps a glass vase to the floor and breaks it. The family is like a busy brain, and the vase is like pain. In this situation, the family is going to be reactive and treat the broken vase as a terrible event. Now picture the family on a two-week vacation. During the second week, someone breaks a vase in the rental condo. The family reacts calmly and does not treat the accident as a major problem. By training your mind to be calm by focusing your attention on your breath, you can train your brain to react calmly to sensory input (pain signals).

MISTAKES TO AVOID

Having shared this breathing exercise with many people, I can tell you the typical mistakes that pain sufferers make when practicing diaphragmatic breathing. After learning the basic instructions and practicing in the psychotherapy session, some patients will go home and plan to practice on a regular basis but forget. Then they have a pain flare-up and suddenly remember, "I have that great new breathing exercise to try. I will start using it now!" And sure enough, they try to do the breathing exercise but find they can hardly concentrate on the breathing and get no benefit from the exercise. If you try to use the breathing exercise only when you have a pain flare-up, it might help, but more likely you will be disappointed. In the worst-case scenario, pain and breathing exercise become linked together. When this occurs, just practicing the breathing will trigger pain.

Learning diaphragmatic breathing is like learning to play the guitar. You could watch a ten-minute YouTube video on how to hold the guitar, play a cord, and strum. It is not that hard. But watching a video for ten minutes or practicing the guitar once or twice does not make you a guitar player. It takes a great deal of daily effort and practice for playing the guitar to feel natural. Learning diaphragmatic breathing is the same. Breathing is not that complicated, but it takes work, practice, and discipline to get all the benefits possible out of the exercise.

PRACTICE MAKES PERMANENT

Rachel enjoyed the practice in the psychology session and thought for sure she would use the exercise at home. That did not happen. The next day, she started her normal routine of getting herself and her kids ready for the day. Before she knew it, she was at work. The workday flew by, and then she was home again with all her usual activities and responsibilities. She fell into bed exhausted, not even thinking about the breathing exercise once.

As she started the next day, she remembered, but not in time to practice in the morning. She decided to take three or four minutes at work to use the exercise there. She actually thought her mind was less busy after the exercise, which helped her respond better to some of the normal challenges she faced. To see if it was just a coincidence, she shut her office door and did another four minutes of breathing. Her mind was very distracted. She could hear her mind say, "This is a waste of time. You have work to do. What if someone sees you? This is not going to help anyway."

She pushed through the noise in her head and kept breathing and redirecting her thoughts. The rest of that day, she still had her fibromyalgia pain, but she functioned better and was a bit more relaxed. Maybe what she experienced the first time was not just by accident.

At home, Rachel began to practice the breathing exercise. She even made diaphragmatic breathing a family event. She and her children would breathe together while lying on their backs in the middle of the living room floor. Her husband was curious, so Rachel gave him some lessons as well. Just before heading off to bed each evening, the two of them would spend a few minutes doing breathing exercises together. The exercise, it turned out, was a nice way to put a barrier up between the busyness of the day and the quietness of the evening. It was not long before Rachel was sleeping a bit better.

14

• • •

PAY ATTENTION TO YOUR BODY

Rachel's struggle with fibromyalgia was related to her spreading pain, sensitivity to normal sensations like her clothing, and sleep problems. Still, she had never met anyone having the symptoms she had, and she felt isolated by her multiple health problems. It did not help that people to whom she tried to explain her health problems looked at her like she was mentally unstable. It hurt her deeply when friends and acquaintances said, "Really? You have chronic pain? But you look fine!" She now avoids telling anyone what is wrong and keeps her struggle to herself.

As she started the pain rehabilitation program, she felt concerned that she would once again get those suspicious, disbelieving looks from the healthcare professionals or get completely impossible advice, such as: "You know, Rachel, research suggests that when people with fibromyalgia start a regular running program, they can cure themselves of chronic pain!" The first time she heard this advice, she said nothing because of how shocked she felt. But now she explains to well-meaning healthcare professionals that she has little strength and finds walking, sitting, and standing painful; she could not run even if she wanted to.

The pain rehabilitation team working with Rachel had better plans for her than starting off with a running program. Rachel first needed some education about chronic pain, and then about sleep hygiene. *Sleep hygiene* is a medical term used to describe the habits that need to be in place for quality sleep to take place. Rachel's sleep hygiene was terrible, and she knew it. She felt trapped by her need to stay alert during the day, her inability to function in the evening without a nap, and her pain throughout the night that interfered with sleep.

During one of the visits with the rehabilitation physician, Rachel's doctor explained the difficult road ahead for her as she corrected her sleep habits. The physician, herself a working mother with a busy professional life, said, "As you make some of the changes that need to be made, you are not going to feel well. Fixing your current habits will further disrupt your sleep and energy levels, but only for a while. Your high levels of caffeine are actually increasing your pain sensitivity. You are in more pain because of all the caffeine, but you are also more alert. Coming off of caffeine will not be easy; you may go through caffeine withdrawal. Not napping when you come home from work will be difficult as well, but that, too, needs to change. You also need to stop watching TV and using your computer at night when you are not sleeping. The good news is that your body needs sleep, wants to sleep, and will sleep. Part of the solution to sleeping better involves getting out of your own body's way so that you can sleep."

Going through all these changes sounded miserable to Rachel. She wanted to blurt out, "Don't you know that I have tried to sleep better? I just cannot sleep! It is not going to happen!" For some reason, she did not say what she was thinking, and instead asked, "Wow. That sounds hard. What am I supposed to do first?" The physician did not single out a specific element of the pain program that would fix the sleep problem but suggested that Rachel would benefit from making many small changes in her life based on what she was learning in physical therapy, occupational therapy, and psychotherapy sessions. All the changes put together would begin to help her not view sleep as a feared enemy. To help Rachel with her difficulty with sleep and pain management, the psychologist introduced the mindfulness body scan.

THE BODY SCAN

Meeting with the psychologist was interesting for Rachel—and not what she expected. She knew all kinds of people who met with psychologists and other types of mental health counselors. Based on their experiences, Rachel was expecting in-depth discussions about her childhood, or explorations into her feelings or sense of self. So far, she had not done anything close to that in the psychology sessions. Instead, she learned a great deal about her mind and body and how they are connected. With each session, she felt that she learned something new that helped her look at her chronic pain a bit differently, which, in a strange way, helped her feel less anxious about all the problems in her life.

It was no surprise when the psychologist started their next session by explaining that they were going to do a body scan exercise. Of course, she had no idea what that was, but she was getting used to being surprised by what she did not know in the pain rehab program.

AWARENESS AND ATTENTION

The body scan was explained as a ten-minute exercise where the attention is directed to different areas of the body, one after another, starting with the feet and moving up to the head. Before the psychologist went into the specifics of how to do the exercise, he wanted Rachel to get the big picture first. The more she understood the concepts and principles behind the body scan, the more likely she would put some energy into practicing the exercise at home.

The psychologist gave Rachel a brief overview of awareness and attention, then he linked those concepts to how the brain produces pain. He started with *attention*—the ability of our mind to shine a spotlight on specific aspects of our experience. He explained that when we go about our day, we generally are not aware of how our attention is being directed. Even without being aware of how attention works, we use our attention to get us through the day. We read, drive, talk, remember, get dressed, call people, turn on devices, and become anxious, bored, and lost in thought all as a function of how our attention is working. Our mind is pointing the spotlight of attention, helping us manage hundreds of tasks every day.

This is where the next concept, *awareness*, comes into the story. We can turn off the automatic pilot and become aware of what our attention is focused on. By being aware, we can notice the actual process of noticing. This probably sounds odd, but you have already done this before. If you have ever had a strange thought randomly run through your mind, you probably said to yourself, "That was weird. Where did that thought come from?" At that moment, you were able to observe your own thoughts.

Observing your thoughts is different than simply thinking that strange, random thought running through your head. You recognize the strange thought is not true or valid.

Think about what happens when pain shows up—the pain gets all of our attention. Take your hands and gradually bring them in front of both of your eyes, stopping about two inches from your face. With your hands in front of your face and your attention on your hands, all you can see is your hands—nothing else. In a similar way, when pain shows up, pain is very powerful at getting all our attention. The spotlight of attention is automatically directed toward pain, and as a result, pain is all that we can notice. Life becomes difficult when all we can see is pain.

By practicing how to focus our attention and notice what is happening, we can learn to have pain move into the background and be just one of the many things we notice. Now take your hands and put them at arm's length in front of you. This is similar to the experience of learning how to accept pain and notice other experiences occurring around you. Life becomes much easier to navigate when all our attention is not focused on pain.

THREE ELEMENTS OF NOTICING

To break the habit of being on automatic pilot, we have the ability to be aware of what is happening in our minds and in the environment around us. Explaining how to be aware is simple, but putting it into practice takes work, just as with the diaphragmatic breathing exercise.

The first element of noticing is intentionally directing your attention toward a target. You can aim your attention like you would aim a flashlight. The second element of noticing is suspending the evaluation the mind typically does when we notice something. The mind is constantly judging, evaluating, and comparing. When practicing how to notice, work on recognizing your mind's tendency to say, "I like that. I don't like that. That is good. That is bad. That feels good. That feels bad." Instead, look at whatever the spotlight of attention is focused on and say nothing about it in your mind. You can practice this part of noticing anytime by looking around the room at different objects and suspending any judgment or evaluation of what you notice.

The final element of noticing is accepting whatever you notice without trying to change it or wishing it to be different. For example, if you happen to focus on an itch on your arm, work at accepting the itch as being there. Try not to evaluate the itch as something good or bad, pleasant or unpleasant, and try not to make yourself more comfortable by relaxing the area or reaching over and scratching it. The only thing you need to do is notice the itch, almost as if you were noticing an itch on someone else's arm. Be curious, accept whatever you notice, and do not evaluate it or try to change it. That is what noticing and paying attention is all about. It is easy to describe but hard to do. In summary, when focusing your attention and noticing, work on these three elements:

- Aim and sustain your attention.
- Suspend judgment. Do not evaluate, describe, or judge what you are noticing.
- Accept what you notice. Do not change or modify what you are noticing.

THE BODY SCAN SCRIPT

This script for completing the body scan exercise can serve as a general guide for completing this exercise. There are many variations and versions of how to complete a body scan, so do not feel that this script needs to be rigidly followed. You might find it useful to use a voice recorder and slowly read the script below with some short pauses in between steps. You can also find a recording of the script on my website: PainRehabSource.com

- Sit upright in a comfortable chair, with both feet on the ground, your back straight, and both arms resting next to your body. Make sure your feet and hands are not touching other parts of your body. If you are lying down, make sure you are flat on your back, with your legs slightly apart and arms and hands not resting anywhere on the body.
- Close your eyes, take a slow deep breath in through the nose, pause for two seconds, and then slowly let the breath out through the mouth. Bring your attention to your stomach as you breathe in and out. (Pause.) Take another slow breath in through the nose, pause for two seconds, then let the breath out through your mouth. (Pause.) Notice the gentle movement of your stomach as you breathe in and out. (Pause.) No effort is needed to breathe. Your body gently brings air into your body breath after breath. (Pause.) Your breath is always there to anchor you and help you settle down.
- Now bring the spotlight of your attention to your feet. Notice what your feet are resting on. Notice the firmness of the floor under your feet. (Pause.) Bring your awareness to any pressure on your feet from socks or shoes you are wearing. Notice

what is in contact with your toes, heels, sides of your feet, and top of your feet. (Pause.) Notice any sensations that are coming from within the feet themselves. (Pause.) You might notice a tingling sensation, warmth, or maybe discomfort. Whatever you notice, allow that sensation to be what it is without evaluating it or trying to change it.

- Now shift your attention to your lower legs. Notice each calf muscle and the shins. As you direct your attention to the lower legs, look for any tension or other sensations that might be in the calf or shins. (Pause.) Notice the surface of your skin and anything touching the skin. If there is any discomfort in your lower leg, just notice where the discomfort is, what direction the discomfort goes, and where it ends. (Pause.)

- Now direct your attention to the upper legs, from your knees to the hips. (Pause.) Notice anything that is touching the surface of the skin along your thighs. (Pause.) Now shift your attention to deep into the muscles of your thighs, and see what you find there. (Pause.) Now direct your attention to the back of your legs. If you are sitting down, notice the weight of your body on the back of your legs. (Pause.) Notice the edge of the chair pressed against your legs. (Pause.) If you are lying down, notice the weight of your legs against the surface you are lying on. (Pause.) As you come across areas of discomfort, allow the sensations to be what they are without evaluating them or trying to change them. (Pause.)

- Now direct the spotlight of attention to your lower back. Notice any discomfort that might be in this area. (Pause.) If there is discomfort, notice where it begins and where it ends. (Pause.) Have your attention shift out toward the hips. (Pause.) Now shift the focus over to the stomach. (Pause.) Notice the gentle movement of the stomach with each breath. (Pause.)

- Bring your awareness to the middle of your back. (Pause.) Notice how the middle of your back is resting against the chair, if you are sitting down, or the floor, bed, or couch, if you are lying down. (Pause.) The muscles that run from the neck to the lower back along the spine often carry tension. See if there are any areas along the spine that are tight or have discomfort. (Pause.) Notice where the tension begins, where it is more intense, and where it ends. (Pause.) Notice the areas of your back where there is no tension or maybe no sensation at all. (Pause.)

- Now bring your attention to your arms. Notice the upper arm, biceps, and triceps. See if you can feel the clothing against your skin in this area. (Pause.) Shift your attention down to your forearms. Notice what your forearms are resting on. (Pause.) Whatever you notice in your forearm, just bring the entire experience into your awareness, even if there is very little to notice.

- Bring your focus to your hands. (Pause.) From the surface of your hands, see if you can sense the temperature of the room you are in. (Pause.) Notice if you can feel the slightest movement of air in the room against the skin of your hands. (Pause.) Notice each individual finger and the change in sensation as you bring your attention fully to your hands. (Pause.)

- Now shift your attention to your shoulders and the base of your neck. (Pause.) This is another area of the body that is often filled with tension and discomfort. Notice where the shoulders and neck have tightness or discomfort. (Pause.) Without judging or evaluating what you are noticing, let the shoulders and neck fill your entire awareness without trying to change and control what you are noticing. (Pause.)

- Now shift your focus to the back of the head. (Pause.) Put the spotlight of attention on the entire surface of your head—notice the forehead, around the ears, the top of the head, and the back of the head. (Pause.) Notice the tension in the skin across your head. (Pause.)

- Now notice your eyes, your eyebrows, and the area below the eyes. (Pause.) Let yourself be aware of how bringing your attention to your eyes allows you to sense changes in the tension around the eyes. (Pause.) You do not need to change any sensations or relax the body. Only notice what happens when you pay attention to your eyes. (Pause.)

- Now bring your attention to your jaw, chin, lips, and face. (Pause.) Notice if there is tension anywhere in your face. (Pause.) Let your entire face come to your awareness, from your chin up to your forehead.

- Gently shift your attention to your nose. (Pause.) Notice the air coming in your nose. Notice that the air is cooler as it enters the nose. (Pause.) As the air leaves your body, notice the warmth of the air as it passes out your nose or your mouth. (Pause.)

- Bring your attention back to your breath. (Pause.) Allow the spotlight of attention to focus in on the gentle movement of your stomach. (Pause.) Take a deeper breath in and hold it for a few seconds. (Pause.) Slowly let the air out. Squeeze your eyes tight. (Pause.) Wiggle your fingers. (Pause.) Now open your eyes.

A TOOL FOR BETTER SLEEP

The impact of the body scan was immediate. Rachel exclaimed, "Practicing the body scan was so strange. I was able to notice my discomfort, but I was not so bothered by it. Then, when I shifted my attention from one area with discomfort to the next, the pain that I was just aware of faded into the background. What happened to it?" Rachel did not realize that the body scan exercise was teaching her pain acceptance and training her brain not to be reactive to the pain she noticed.

As Rachel was led through this exercise with the psychologist for the first time, she had great difficulty staying awake for the entire ten minutes. The more she tried to focus her attention, the more her mind and body relaxed and drifted toward sleep. The psychologist explained that he has had many sleep-deprived pain patients fall sound asleep during body scan exercises. He went on to suggest that Rachel specifically practice immediately before going to bed each night. Many patients have reported that the body scan was one of the first steps they took toward sleeping better at night.

Rachel was willing to try anything, even doing a body scan before bed. On the first night of doing the exercise on her own, she noticed how busy and disrupted her mind was when attempting to focus her attention. Time after time she needed to redirect her attention back to the task at hand. She also struggled with trying to notice the discomfort in her body without changing or evaluating it. She thought she was not doing well with the body scan, but she rolled over, fell asleep, and rested deeply for a few hours before waking up again. Since the body scan helped her fall asleep so easily, she used the exercise again to get relaxed and reduce the irritation and burning sensations. It took several days of practice, but in time, she was able to sleep for longer periods of time and feel more rested in the morning.

15

● ● ●

REDUCE MUSCLE TENSION

After the first few weeks in the pain rehabilitation program, David began to see small changes take place with his lower back and leg pain. He had not been able to tolerate bending, walking, or standing for any length of time for the past two years. Now he could go for five minutes three times a day and do simple exercises and stretches. This was progress he never thought he would make. Still, David was impatient and wanted to see even more change.

The pressure he experienced from his injury, chronic pain, and difficulty of being out of work, all worked together to increase David's level of stress and muscle tension throughout his body. Even while he was in the rehabilitation program, his back and neck were becoming stiff and sore. He was having headaches more frequently, and it was difficult for him to relax well enough to sleep deeply.

When he mentioned some of the struggles with sleep and soreness to his psychologist, she asked him what he thought might be happening. David honestly did not know. He did not see a connection between his stress and his increased discomfort. He actually thought the pain rehab program was just too much for him and wondered if he should back off from the program or even take a break from it altogether.

Then he recalled what all the team members in the pain program said: "Your brain wants to protect you. It will protect you by sending you to your bed, closing blinds, turning off the lights, and shutting the door. Your brain is not trying to heal you. If you listen to your brain's rules, you will not get better."

The psychologist then asked David if some of the stress associated with his pain and life circumstances might be influencing the amount of physical tension he has in his back and neck. Once again, he was not certain but doubted it.

The psychologist handed David a small plastic thermometer to put between his thumb and index finger. As David put the finger thermometer in place, the psychologist asked David to describe some of his most recent financial struggles arising from his unemployment status. After three minutes of talking, David and the psychologist looked at the temperature on the finger thermometer, which was eighty degrees Fahrenheit (twenty-six degrees Celsius). The psychologist then wanted to know what was happening with the tension in his back and neck. Not surprisingly, a great deal of tension and the start of a headache had shown up while he was talking about his financial stress.

David was not sure what the connection was between the temperature in his hands and the tension in his back and neck. The psychologist didn't answer, asking David to hold on to his questions until after trying another relaxation exercise called *progressive muscle relaxation* (PMR). She was confident that after she explained PMR and practiced the relaxation exercise with David, David would see a change in his hand temperature and have reduced tension in his back and neck. She felt that if David personally experienced the mind-body connection using the PMR, he would be more convinced that his thoughts, body temperature, and muscle tension were all connected. He was not going to be convinced by just an explanation.

MUSCLE TENSION AND STRESS

To understand how muscle tension and stress build up, picture yourself behind the wheel of a car driving from a rural, quiet area toward a major city like Chicago or New York. You start your journey using slow, two-lane county roads and then join a larger state highway. As you get closer to the city, you leave the state highway for massive interstate highways. Far from your slow county roads, you now are in the middle of a five-lane highway with several semi-trucks blocking your view.

Now add two more elements to this picture—it is dark and pouring rain. For most people, this type of driving is stressful. If you are anything like me, your shoulders and back start getting tense. When driving in these conditions, a knot develops in my muscles that feels like someone is pushing their knuckle right into my back. It hurts!

In this stressful situation, not only will the muscles become tight throughout the back, but there is actually a reduction in blood flow to those tight muscles. This reduced blood flow is significant because the muscles build up lactic acid as they remain tight. As the lactic acid builds up, it is not removed quickly because of the reduced blood flow. This combination of increased lactic acid and reduced blood flow adds to the pain we experience with muscle tension.

Progressive muscle relaxation helps us bypass the automatic control that the brain has over those tense muscles.[1.] When we are under stress, the autonomic nervous system is in charge of what happens to muscles throughout the body, preparing them for action. The body gets ready to fight, flee, or to hide, increasing the muscle tension in the back. Because this physical response is automatic, I cannot simply say to my back, shoulder, and neck muscles, "Hey, muscles! Stop being tense! Relax down to the level of tension I feel on a beach vacation." It would be great if I could make my muscles respond like that, but they simply cannot. It would be just as hard to tell your heart rate to instantly go from 140 beats per minute to 65 beats per minute.

BYPASS AUTOMATIC CONTROL

While we cannot consciously change muscle tension caused by stress, we can bypass the automatic control that the brain has over muscle tension. When our muscles are completely relaxed, the tension level is low. When we are under stress, the tension level is in the medium range, but if we intentionally flex or tighten the muscles as hard as possible, the tension level is high.

When we flex our muscles and then relax them—as we do in PMR—the tension in the muscles will go back down to the low level of tension. If I were driving my car toward Chicago on the busy, congested highways, I would notice the tension in my back and neck. After noticing the tension, I could go through the progressive muscle relaxation (PMR) exercise (while driving) and bring the tension in the muscles back down into the low range.

PMR is portable and easy to use. Sitting in meetings,

standing in long lines, or traveling long distances are all opportunities to use PMR.

As David was introduced to the PMR exercise, he was not too convinced he even needed an exercise like this. He did not have a strong connection in his mind between stress, his thinking, and his muscle tension. All he was aware of was soreness, stiffness, and pain developing in his back and neck. He was not paying attention to his stress or what he was thinking about. He was suspicious that his back and neck were hurting more because of doing physical exercises and stretches associated with the pain rehabilitation program.

David's lack of awareness of how his stress impacted his tension and pain was not a concern to the psychologist. She knew the PMR exercise would be helpful to him regardless of what he thought about stress or even the PMR exercise. She explained that he should not expect the exercise to be relaxing. Completing the exercise would take energy, concentration, and using a lot of muscles. The exercise would have to be completed before David would feel a general sense of relaxation throughout the body.

PROGRESSIVE MUSCLE RELAXATION SCRIPT

Completing the PMR exercise will take about ten minutes and can be completed while sitting in a chair or lying down. The following are the four principles to keep in mind while practicing:

- As you begin to tense a muscle group, slowly inhale. The tensing phase can last from four to ten seconds. As you release the tension in the muscles, breathe out slowly. Count to four as you tense the muscles and count again to four as you gradually release the tension.

- Gradually tense and release the tension in the muscles. Picture the tension in the muscles slowly flowing out of the muscles down toward the ground as you release the tension.

- When tensing the muscles, be careful not to let the peak tension reach the level of pain or cramping. If you feel your muscles begin to cramp, slowly back off on the level of tension. Getting clearance from your doctor or physical therapist to do this exercise is important.

- Daily practice is needed to benefit from this exercise. Practicing PMR mid- or late afternoon can be helpful since that is when muscle tension is often highest during the day. Evening practice just before going to sleep can help significantly with falling asleep.

- You can read the following PMR script out loud and record the dialog so you can practice more easily. You can also find a recording of this script on my website: PainRehabSource.com.

- Sit upright in a comfortable chair with both feet on the ground, your back straight, and both arms resting next to your body. If you are lying down, make sure you are flat on your back, with your legs slightly apart and arms and hands not resting anywhere on your body.

- Close your eyes, take a slow deep breath in through the nose, pause for two seconds, and then slowly let the breath out through the mouth. Bring your attention to your stomach as you breathe in and out. (Pause.) Take another slow breath in through the nose, pause for two seconds, then let the breath out through your mouth. (Pause.)

- Take a few more breaths and with each breath out, imagine the tension in your body flowing out of you. Picture the tension like water flowing down toward the ground.
- Bring your attention to your eyes. In just a moment, you will squeeze your eyes tightly shut and inhale slowly on a count of four when I say, "Begin." When I say, "Release," you will breathe out on a count of four and picture all the tension around your eyes flowing away.
- Begin: one, two, three, four. Release: one, two, three, four. Your eyes feel warm and relaxed. (Pause.)
- Keeping your eyes closed, slowly begin to raise your eyebrows as high as you can, tensing your entire forehead and scalp. Slowly breathe in as you begin to tense.
- Begin: one, two, three, four. Release: one, two, three, four. Your forehead feels loose and relaxed. (Pause.)
- Now slowly begin to smile with your entire face, keeping your eyes closed.
- Begin: one, two, three, four. Release: one, two, three, four. Notice all the tension leaving your face as it becomes relaxed. (Pause.)
- Now focus on your neck muscles. Slowly draw your chin in and tighten your neck muscles.
- Begin: one, two, three, four. Release: one, two, three, four. Feel the warmth come to your neck as the tension leaves. (Pause.)
- Now gradually lift your shoulders up toward your ears and then tighten your shoulders from the outer shoulder to the base of your neck.

- Begin: one, two, three, four. Release: one, two, three, four. Your shoulders feel loose, limp, and relaxed. (Pause.)
- Turn your hands so your palms face upward, and slowly close your fingers to make a fist. Roll your fists toward your forearms. Bring tension to your biceps and forearms like you are carrying a heavy load of wood.
- Begin: one, two, three, four. Release: one, two, three, four. Notice the tension leaving your arms, which now feel loose and relaxed.
- Turn your hands so the palms are facing down. Spread out your fingers, stretching them away from each other, opening your hands as wide as possible.
- Begin: one, two, three, four. Release: one, two, three, four. Your hands now feel loose and limp as the tension flows away.
- Bring both hands up to your chest, place your palms against each other, and press your hands against each other, bringing tension to your entire chest.
- Begin: one, two, three, four. Release: one, two, three, four. (Pause.)
- Now focus on your back. Slowly bring your shoulders back, and then draw your shoulder blades toward each other, slightly arching your back, tensing your entire back.
- Begin: one, two, three, four. Release: one, two, three, four. Feel all the tension leave your back, flowing down toward the ground.
- Bring your attention to your stomach. Tighten all of your stomach muscles, including the muscles of your lower back.
- Begin: one, two, three, four. Release: one, two, three, four. (Pause.)

- Now focus on your upper legs. From your knees to your hips, slowly begin to tighten your thighs, the back of your legs, and your bottom. Breathe in as you begin to tense.
- Begin: one, two, three, four. Release: one, two, three, four. Your legs feel loose, limp, and relaxed. (Pause.)
- Now lift your toes up toward your shins and push your heels down. Slowly bring tension to the calf muscles and shins.
- Begin: one, two, three, four. Release: one, two, three, four. Feel the tension leave your lower legs, flowing down toward the ground.
- Curl your toes down toward the bottom of your feet, tensing both feet.
- Begin: one, two, three, four. Release: one, two, three, four. Your feet feel warmer, relaxed, and limp. (Pause.)
- Take a slow deep breath in through the nose, hold your breath for two seconds, and then slowly let the breath out through the mouth. Bring your attention to your stomach as you breathe in and out. Inhale again and notice with each breath out the weight of tension throughout your body flowing away. Picture tension leaving your body like water flowing from you down into the ground.
- Squeeze your eyes shut tightly and then relax your eyes. Take a deep breath in, wiggle your fingers, and open your eyes.
- You can also find a recording of the PMR script on my website: PainRehabSource.com

MAKING THE CONNECTION

As David went through the PMR exercise with the psychologist, he was more focused on doing all the steps correctly and was not sure if there was much benefit from the exercise. Then the psychologist handed him the finger thermometer again. During the PMR exercise, his skin temperature had gone up eight degrees, and the tension in his shoulders reduced.

During his next appointment the following week, he reported that with regular practice he was successful in becoming more relaxed. He also discovered something unexpected—his back and neck muscles seemed to have less tension in them throughout the day. The PMR exercise gave him a method to notice the difference between relaxed and tense muscles. It had never been hard for him to recognize the soreness and stiffness, but now he was aware of the actual tension in the muscles.

As he made the connection between physical tension and his sore body, it was not hard for him to notice when he often became tense. Every morning, he was always busy with making plans, going to medical visits, and doing chores. But in the afternoon, he would sit in his recliner and start to think. The more he sat and thought about his life, future, and current financial situation, the worse he felt emotionally and physically. It was during this time of the day his muscles would become tense.

He always thought of depression as some kind of weakness and had no interest in identifying himself as depressed. As David talked about how the tension built up each afternoon, the psychologist suggested that acknowledging that he was upset was not a weakness, but a sign of strength. By accepting his feelings, he would become more willing to look at his stress and the weight he felt on his shoulders.

The mind-body connection was made; David could connect the dots between the neck and back pain with the muscle tension and his discouraging life circumstances. The connection in his mind did not solve the problems he was facing, but it did reduce the tension and discomfort he was experiencing in his back and neck. He began to discuss his stress and feelings with his wife, his parents, and a few close friends. These open discussions helped David find hope for handling the problems and pressure he was facing. He was no longer carrying the heavy load alone, and his thoughts were not as upsetting when they went through his mind.

16

• • •

OVERCOMING
THE FEAR OF MOVEMENT

A barrier for many pain sufferers is the fear of movement—if they walk, stand, reach, bend, step, or twist, it hurts. The fear of movement is understandable. Pain is the brain trying to protect us. It tells us to stop moving or doing things that are going to aggravate an already bad situation. Our fear of movement, therefore, is a protective response of the brain, but it also creates a problem. If we listen to the advice our brain is giving us, we would never get out of bed in the morning.

We often fail to realize how important movement is to healthy functioning. When we are in pain, we can easily cut back on movement, not realizing the negative consequences of what can happen as a result. For example, if a healthy person with no specific pain issues or injuries stays in bed for hours both day and night, he or she will soon be sick. Here are some of the changes that will occur:

- Reduced cardiac output (the heart pumps less blood)
- Reduced blood volume
- Muscle shrinkage

- Reduced bone density and strength
- Less balance when standing
- Increased dizziness and lightheadedness
- Increased pain with movement
- More elastic veins, making it difficult for blood to return to the heart
- Increased negative mood

By just staying in bed, on a couch, or in a recliner for days at a time, a healthy person turns into a sick person with chronic pain. To demonstrate this fact, medical researchers in 2004 examined the prescription of bed rest for acute back pain. While bed rest is not the recommended course of treatment for low back pain, many doctors still prescribe it as a part of their treatment plans.[1.] Patients with acute low back pain who followed medical advice to stay in bed even for only four days were 32 percent more likely to develop chronic pain and needed more medications to treat their pain than those patients who received treatment that included movement.

THE PROTECTION CYCLE

If you have ever slipped on ice or lost your footing on carpeted stairs and landed hard on your back, you know what it is like to suddenly experience pain. After the injury took place, you were probably very careful for several weeks to avoid slipping or falling again. Every time you saw a slippery patch on the sidewalk or approached carpeted stairs, you braced yourself and stepped very cautiously. Being self-protective after an injury is natural, but avoiding activities altogether is taking protection too far and can lead to unexpected problems.

When we experience ongoing pain, our brain tells us, "Sit down. Lie down. Don't move." If we guard ourselves and restrict our activity so that we stop exercising, walking, swimming, or stretching, we will end up deconditioned, which is another way of saying we get out of shape. When we are deconditioned, three problems will occur with our muscles:

- First, the muscles become weaker and everyday activities become harder. Just walking around the house or up a flight of stairs will be difficult and tiring.
- Second, the muscles will not work as they should and will complain when used, causing spasms, cramps, twitches, and electric-shock sensations. Once the muscles are dysfunctional, just using the muscles during normal activities will lead to additional pain. Daily activities such as brushing teeth, combing hair, and getting dressed become increasingly painful and difficult.
- Third, with limited use of our hands, arms, legs, neck, and back, our joints will become stiffer, making even simple movements uncomfortable.

Fortunately, the protection cycle can be broken. Research of individuals with chronic pain has repeatedly shown that activities such as strength training, riding a stationary bike, walking, or exercise in a pool are excellent ways to immediately improve a person's functioning and break the protection cycle.[2.] As a person then continues with exercise, the positive results last, and the improvements will continue.

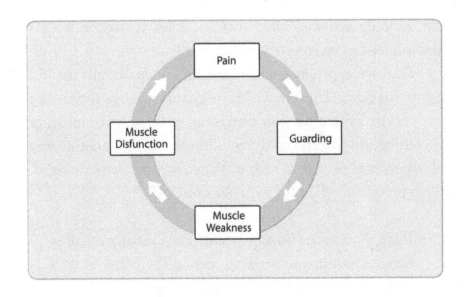

FEAR OF MOVEMENT

When a person falls into the protection cycle trap, it can be a hard climb back to being physically active. If this describes you, know that there is hope and that the struggle that you face to get moving again is going to be worth it. The biggest hurdle you have to face is not being physically weak—your greatest enemy is the fear of movement. Your brain is quick to learn what causes pain and then reminds you that you will hurt if you are going to engage in some activity associated with pain. We need to break the mental connection between what your brain has learned in the past (movement equals pain) and create a new connection so the brain learns that movement equals healing and recovery.

Some of the key elements to breaking the connection between movement and pain were covered in chapter 11 when we discussed danger-in-me (DIM) and safety-in-me (SIM) messages.

The first step in making a new connection in your brain will require carefully examining your DIMs and SIMs, working to build up good information, hope, and medical research about movement and healing in order to overcome the false learning that has already taken place. Your brain does not change easily, and new habits take time to form.

You will also want to work on accepting your pain. When you turn toward what is difficult and threatening with a sense of willingness and openness, you interfere with your brain's ability to produce fear. We will discuss pain acceptance in greater detail later in the book, but the key idea here is that by accepting pain, you actually turn down the fear volume in your brain. Fear is associated with the behavior of running away, avoiding, and hiding. Accepting pain means that we create a space for difficulty and discomfort without trying to control it or avoid it. While acceptance might sound like an unusual approach to pain, pain acceptance is central to effective pain management and to move toward a life that is rich and meaningful, even with ongoing problems with pain.

While you are working on accepting pain, you should also work on accepting the fear and anxiety associated with pain. Fear and anxiety are unpleasant emotions. These emotions are very good at getting us to stop, change directions, and do whatever we can to avoid anxiety and fear. When we attempt to manage fear and anxiety by trying to control or run away from them, we end up with more fear and anxiety. In the next section of the book, we will discuss how acceptance actually works, but you can begin working on accepting negative emotions by evaluating your current efforts to control fear and anxiety and asking yourself these questions:

Have my efforts to control fear and anxiety eliminated these emotions from my life? Were my efforts successful?

What have my efforts to control fear and anxiety cost me? How many events and good things have I missed out on because of my fear of not knowing what would happen with my pain or anxiety?

When we come face to face with the truth that our own efforts to manage negative emotions have not worked, we become more open to trying other approaches for dealing with chronic pain. An approach outlined in the third section of the book involves three main elements:

- Learn to let go.
- Learn to be present.
- Learn to move forward.

You'll battle with different thoughts and internal struggles as you begin moving, stretching, walking, and strength training. Your mind is going to be busy being upset about the changes you are making and will create a whole host of catastrophic, negative, fear-filled statements. Here are some that you can expect to hear your mind say:

- I am going to make things worse if I exercise.
- I cannot stand the pain.
- I am going to hurt myself if I move too much.
- The pain is going to be terrible when I exercise.
- If I make the pain worse, the pain will never go away.
- I tried to exercise before and failed. This is not going to help.

- I am too out of shape to do anything. People are going to laugh.

When these fears start acting up, rather than trying to push the fear and thoughts away, try to view these thoughts as normal brain activity. You could say to yourself, "Thank you, brain, for your input! I can always count on you for the bad news. I know you are only trying to help." The noise of these negative statements does not represent what you are all about or define who you are as a person—it is just noise.

WHERE TO BEGIN

Regardless of your pain condition, you need to be evaluated by a healthcare professional and receive approval to begin a fitness program. It would not be possible to outline one general program that applies to everyone facing problems with chronic pain, but the basics of what is covered in most conditioning and training programs will be outlined. I will also suggest specific resources that will be helpful to you and your specific pain condition.

There are four basic elements of a fitness program for chronic pain rehabilitation: (1) warm-up, (2) endurance exercise, (3) strength exercise, and (4) cooldown. Maybe you have tried an exercise plan in the past or had a negative experience with physical therapy and found that physical activity was simply too painful. To avoid having fitness only being associated with pain, many people must begin with just the warm-up phase.

- The warm-up involves getting your body and your muscles ready to move. At its most basic level, warming up might be just applying a heating pad to different areas of your body. For most people, warming up involves gentle stretching, swinging the arms up and down or in a circle, marching in place, and gently moving the neck, shoulders, arms, hands, back, legs, hips, and feet through simple range-of-motion exercises to get the blood flowing to these areas.

- Endurance exercise, also called *aerobic exercise*, uses the large muscles of the body to increase the heart rate. There is no substitute for doing endurance exercise on a regular basis. For some pain sufferers, this exercise may just be five minutes of slow walking. When we regularly engage in endurance exercise, happy chemicals in the brain (endorphins) are released.

- In our discussion of the gate theory of the spine, you will remember that endorphins travel down the spine and help block sensory information coming up the spine to the brain. In short, exercise helps block pain. It also helps to improve mood and motivation. Regular aerobic exercise also reduces the risk of a wide variety of health problems, including cancer, diabetes, arthritis, depression, heart disease, and obesity.

- If you are not sure where to start, stationary exercise bikes are low impact but effective at increasing your heart rate. Keep in mind to exercise only for five minutes as you begin. Other exercises, such as walking, jogging, biking, swimming, dancing, or using a rowing machine, are all good options to explore. Work to have five to six days a week of endurance exercise in your schedule. With all of these exercises, follow the principles of pacing. Do five or ten minutes of exercise, followed by rest, and then more exercise. Stay out of the pain zone, but limit your time in the discomfort zone. Work toward getting your endurance activities up to thirty minutes per day. Getting up to thirty minutes may take several weeks.

- Strength training helps put your muscles to use. A basic principle for healthy living is to recognize that our bodies are made for work. If we do not use our muscles, they will shrink in size (atrophy). Without real physical work, such as lifting, carrying, chopping wood, or strength training, our muscles lose function, which leads to increased pain.

- Unused, out-of-shape muscles have cramps, electric shocks, tightness, soreness, and achiness, all just from deconditioning. If you have chronic pain, consult with a physical therapist or occupational therapist who is knowledgeable about your condition to learn safe ways to begin strength training.

- Some pain sufferers simply start exercising by just squeezing a small exercise ball or clay putty to strengthen their weak hands. Fitness bands made of rubber are also helpful for gentle strengthening when used properly. Working on balance is also important as you recover from chronic pain.

- Keep in mind that physical therapy practices worldwide are kept busy because of patients who have injuries from fitness programs that repeatedly have participants do similar exercises to the point of exhaustion. Variety is the key to any strength training program. Work at putting strength training into your schedule three or four times per week.

- Cooldown exercises are important for ensuring proper recovery after exercise. There needs to be a slowing down of activity, such as gently walking, stretching, or going through range-of-motion exercises to help the body recover from the exercise. The cooldown period might include putting heating pads or ice packs on different areas of your body. Massaging your muscles with your hands or with a tennis ball can also help your muscles recover. Professional and serious amateur athletes benefit from a range of post-workout massages using foam or pliability rollers, and these tools can be great for pain patients as well. Foam rollers help reduce soreness and speed the recovery of muscles after exercise.

COMMITTED ACTION

I have worked with people who have not exercised in twenty years, as well as top athletes who have lost thirty pounds (thirteen kilograms) of muscle after a serious injury. The effort that it takes to get moving again is mostly mental, not physical. We put up barriers to resist change and experience depressed moods and low motivation. This is not a good combination. Here are some reasons your brain will give you about why you should not start working out:

- I do not like exercising alone.
- I do not want others to see me.
- I am overweight and look bad.
- It is too cold, too hot, too wet, or too dry outside.
- It is too much work.
- I do not have the time.
- It will take too much time to regain what I lost.

These statements are just noise in your brain, and there is no point in trying to talk yourself out of the noise. The word machine in your head will always produce these statements and more like them. The closer you get to actually exercising, the louder the noise of these negative messages will get. Besides learning to accept the dialog running through your brain, you will also need to do one more important thing—commit yourself to taking action.

If you approach exercise with the intention to wait and see if you like to exercise before you commit, your chances of following through with a fitness program will be low. Lasting change takes solid commitment before you start. Committed action and acceptance go hand in hand with each other. If you accept the struggle of moving forward, you will also accept that it will be hard to change and push through the difficulties of starting an exercise program. But if you do not accept the challenge and do not make a total commitment to change, then struggle, discouragement, and discomfort will register as signs that you should quit, and you probably will.

If you do start and then quit, that is okay. The next time you start, before you begin your fitness program, write down your plan, share your plan openly with others, get accountability, and make a commitment. Starting a fitness plan with this approach will ensure your success.

There is a series of books written by the physical therapist Robin McKenzie on how to do safe exercises and stretches for different areas of the body, including the neck, shoulders, knees, and back. It is a very good approach to working with people who have chronic pain. Ask about these books at your local book dealer, or order them online. They can be a great help to you in your own pain rehabilitation process.

STEP THREE

DEVELOP EMOTIONAL FLEXIBILITY

Health is a great blessing, but the moment you make health one of your main, direct objects you start becoming a crank and imagining there is something wrong with you. You are only likely to get health provided you want other things more—food, games, work, fun, open air.

—C. S. Lewis (1898–1963)

Every person struggling with chronic pain should ask themselves why it is important for them to learn how to manage pain. If your only answer to this vital question is that you would like to have less pain, then you will need to dig deeper, think harder. What would you do if you were not so affected by pain? What do you want to do with a healthier mind and body? As you begin to get a clear picture of your future, you have the beginnings of real hope for change.

Becoming emotionally flexible involves three key elements: (1) letting go of what is in the way, (2) staying connected to the present moment, and (3) moving toward what is important. These three principles will help us get untangled from the thoughts, emotions, sensations, and self-concepts that keep us trapped in a cycle of distress and short-term relief. When looking at how we deal with chronic pain, we often fall prey to the appeal of short-term relief rather than to push through and do the rewarding work of moving forward. This third section of the book will walk you through the steps you need to start living a life that is full of meaning and vitality.

17

• • •

THE STRUGGLE CYCLE

N ancy received a call from her daughter on a Monday evening, reminding her that her granddaughter's fifth birthday
party was set for Saturday at noon. Nancy took a deep breath
and said for what seemed like the hundredth time, "Well, I don't
know for sure if I'll make it. I would like to come, but I will see
what I am like on Saturday. I will sure try." Nancy's daughter
was used to this kind of response from her mom, and Nancy
could sense her irritation. Just getting this call from her daughter
increased Nancy's pain; she hated to let so many people down.

WHAT IS SUFFERING?

Most people with chronic pain describe suffering as the constant misery caused by pain. When Nancy thought about
missing out on one more important event like her granddaughter's
birthday, she pointed to pain as the source of the problem. Pain
was getting in her way, making her life miserable and causing
her to suffer. She wanted to go to the party, but the pain would
keep her stuck at home. She hoped to someday have more
control over her pain.

Who would not want to have control over their pain? Control over pain is why millions of medications are sold every year and why surgeries are offered as solutions to misery and suffering. We all seem to picture a good life as one that is pain-free and happy, and the way to get there is to gain control over pain and negative emotions.

When people describe their years of struggle with pain to me, I ask whether their efforts to control pain have brought relief and long-term results. This is exactly what Nancy's psychologist did. He asked, "So, Nancy, have you had to say no to parties, family gatherings, weddings, graduations, and things like that in the past because of your migraines and headaches?" Yes, of course, she has had to say no to these events. Then the psychologist asked an unexpected question about the effectiveness of her approach to managing pain, "Has it helped?"

Nancy looked at the psychologist with a confused expression. She then asked, "What do you mean, has it helped? I've avoided going to these events because I might end up halfway through and have a bad headache. Or if I woke up in the morning with a headache, I could not imagine going anywhere. What else was I supposed to do?"

The psychologist acknowledged her point and replied, "Think about this for a minute. Has avoiding important meaningful events helped you get rid of your headaches in the past twenty years?" Nancy admitted that avoiding events had not helped, so the psychologist added, "I wonder if the suffering you have experienced has come at least in part from the effort and struggle you have put into trying to control your migraines. It sounds like you have a number of losses in your life from missing out on what is important to you."

This was a new thought for Nancy. She had never considered her efforts to control her pain as a problem. Her immediate reaction to this new thought was sadness. As she sat with the feelings of loss that were coming up, the best she could do to keep her tears back was to ask once again what she was supposed to do.

The psychologist gave an interesting definition of suffering, one that Nancy had never heard of before. He explained that suffering is trying to fix something that cannot be fixed. All the attempts to control chronic pain actually leads to a greater degree of suffering, more than the suffering from the pain itself. Nancy could see that trying to control things she could not control was part of her life. She worried about her pain, planned her life around her pain, stopped living her life in order to control and avoid pain, but in the end, had the same pain, despite all of her efforts.

After a moment of silence and reflection, Nancy asked, "This Saturday, I do not know if I am going to have a headache or migraine. How can I commit to going to the birthday party? Is that what you are saying I should do—go to the party even with a bad headache?"

The psychologist redirected the question back to Nancy, "What would it look like if you woke up on Saturday morning, had the beginnings of a headache, and still made a decision to go to the party?"

Nancy replied, "Well, I could go to the party with a headache, but it might get worse."

Once again, the psychologist wanted Nancy to see the core of her struggle and said, "What would it be like going to a party with a headache? What if you went and it got worse?"

Nancy blurted out, "If I go, I cannot control it! How could I stay if I have a headache?"

The moment she said this, the little light bulb turned on in her mind, and she said, "Oh, I get it. If I stay home, I am trying to control and avoid the headache. In twenty years, staying home has never worked. I still get headaches and migraines, even at home. If I go to the party, I will not be able to control pain there either."

The psychologist asked, "What would it be like for you to go to the party? What is important about being there?"

Now the tears came to Nancy's eyes as she answered, "I would be a part of my family's life—my granddaughter's life. I would see their smiles myself, not just pictures from someone who was there. That is very important to me."

The psychologist sat in silence with Nancy as she felt the years of loss in her life. She thought about all the events, family memories, and precious moments she must have missed out on by staying at home. The psychologist then explained, "Suffering is trying to control what we cannot control. Our efforts to control and avoid pain adds to the pain we already experience in our lives. Control adds to our suffering. This is why accepting what we cannot change is one of the most important steps we can take when faced with chronic pain or difficult thoughts and emotions." Nancy thought this sounded good, but how was she ever going to learn to accept pain? She hated pain. Pain was her enemy, and she had no interest in making friends with pain.

PAYING ATTENTION

For Nancy to change from being stuck in her struggle with pain to moving forward with her life, she needed to learn about letting go, staying present, and moving toward what was important to her. To help with the process of teaching these principles, the psychologist drew a picture with one vertical line and one horizontal line, with the two lines intersecting exactly in the middle. The horizontal line had an arrowhead on each end, one pointing to the left, and the other to the right. He then drew a circle where the two lines intersected in the middle.

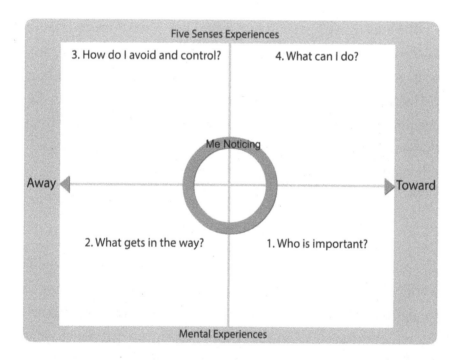

The psychologist was using a visual tool called the Matrix. The Matrix is used in acceptance and commitment therapy (ACT therapy) to help people notice what is happening in their

lives and help them become more flexible and moving in a direction that is important to them.[1.] As Nancy heard this brief
description of the Matrix, she thought of her sadness regarding
what she had missed out on in life and the desire she had to be
engaged in life again. She wondered if the Matrix would help
her sort out her problems and get her moving forward.

THE OUTSIDE WORLD

Before we continue with Nancy's story, let's take a closer look at
the Matrix diagram. You might want to draw one for yourself and
use the Matrix as you go through this and the following chapters.

The area above the solid horizontal line is what we can notice
in the outside world. We can notice the things we smell, see,
hear, taste, and touch. We can also notice what we do and how
we interact with others. When we are describing what is in the
outside world, we can use a video camera to record everything
that our five senses experience and the actions we take. The outside world is always there, no matter what we are doing.

THE INSIDE WORLD

The area below the horizontal line represents the private inner
world of your mind. You can shift your attention to notice
thoughts, feelings, sensations, memories, self-concepts, values,
desires, and wants. With your inside world, you can notice what
it is like when you are engaged in meaningful activities, doing
what is important to you. You can notice satisfaction, pleasure,
and good feelings. You can also notice things that make it hard
to enjoy what is important to you and how you react when those

experiences and thoughts occur. When unpleasant memories, negative thoughts, painful sensations, and difficult emotions show up, you can notice how you instinctively want to pull away from all of that distress. All of these pleasant and unpleasant things take place out of view of others because they are in your private, inner world. The inside world is different than the five senses—only you can notice what is in your own mind.

ME NOTICING

The circle in the middle of the diagram represents your ability to pay attention to different parts of your experience. When I focus my attention on where I am sitting right now, I can use my five senses and see different objects on my desk, smell the air in the room, hear several near and far away sounds, sense a variety of sensations against my skin, and even become aware of the taste in my mouth.

The experience of directing my attention outward is very different than when I direct my attention inward and focus on the thoughts that I have about being hungry, memories of what happened yesterday, emotions about family news I recently heard, and tasks that I would like to accomplish before the end of the day. As I direct my attention inward to the privacy of my mind, I see several negative things as well, including worrisome thoughts, self-judgments, blame, dark predictions of what will happen, memories of past losses, painful physical sensations, and expectations of disappointment in the future. When we put the spotlight of attention on the private world of the mind, we see a complicated mix of realistic, distorted, hopeful, dark, and discouraging thoughts and inner experiences.

WHAT AND WHO IS IMPORTANT

The two arrowheads on the horizontal line point to the right and the left. To the right is the word "Toward" and to the left is the word "Away." These two directions represent two aspects of our experience that we can notice. We can notice what our personal experience is like when we are moving toward what is important. When we move toward what is important, we notice a sense of satisfaction, meaning, and purpose. As we live out our values and move toward what is important, we feel good—not because everything turns out well and life is easy, but because we are living in line with what we believe is important. Nancy loves her children and grandchildren. She values close relationships, intimacy, and adventure. The time she spends with her friends and family is rewarding and meaningful to her.

WHAT GETS IN OUR WAY

The arrow to the left represents what shows up in our lives that makes it hard to move toward what is important to us. When Nancy moves toward what is important to her and plans to join her family on the many activities she missed out on over the years, a number of thoughts, memories, emotions, and sensations start to show up, including:

- Memories of past family vacations that were miserable for her.
- Predictions of how bad this trip will be for her.
- Anxiety about not having control over the pain.
- Pain that is happening right now.

- Physical tension in her neck and shoulders.
- Anger about how people respond to her in pain.
- Anxiety and sadness about disappointing the people she loves.
- Fear of being in the car and having pain flare up.
- Anxiety about not knowing where she will be sleeping.
- The self-concept of her being weak and sickly.
- Feelings of loneliness from not being understood.
- Anxiety and sadness about missing out and staying home instead.
- The thought that she has to stop the pain with any means possible.

All of these thoughts, feelings, memories, self-concepts, and sensations show up and have one main effect on Nancy—they create discomfort. The technical definition of discomfort is "a yucky feeling." We do not like yucky feelings. The Away arrow side of the Matrix represents what we want to do when tension and discomfort show up in our lives; we want to pull away from the discomfort and yucky feelings.

THE TRAP

We want to move toward what is important to us, but when something shows up that makes it hard to go forward, we often pull away and move in the opposite direction of where we really want to go. Picture a rabbit running through a neighborhood early in the morning. It notices that someone planted a small garden and immediately becomes excited. The rabbit values good food, a healthy breakfast, and a quick, efficient meal. As it hops toward the garden, the rabbit notices the inner sense of excitement and satisfaction. The rabbit is energized by moving toward what is important to it.

The rabbit arrives in the backyard where the garden is located and suddenly notices that it is not alone. In the backyard is a large, muscular dog sitting on the back porch, without any collar or chain. The dog sees the rabbit. Suddenly, the rabbit notices a new sensation—a yucky feeling. This yucky feeling is very strong and unpleasant, and the rabbit wonders how to get rid of its terrible discomfort. It decides to turn around and run in the opposite direction of the garden. The dog chases after, but not quickly enough. Upon escaping from the dog, the rabbit notices the yucky feeling is gradually going away. It also realizes something more important. It is now far away from where it wanted to be. Yes, running away reduced the bad feelings, but it also eliminated the sense of satisfaction and pleasure it had when it was in the garden.

Nancy's experience mirrors the rabbit's. When Nancy noticed her upsetting thoughts, feelings, memories, and sensations throughout the day, the pain seemed to increase. Without thinking about her options, she did what she always did—she automatically reacted just like the rabbit did with the dog. Her instinct was to reduce the tension by trying to get rid of the yucky feelings. She couldn't run away, of course, but she could reach into her purse and look for some medication to lessen her pain or take an antacid tablet to settle her stomach, which was getting upset from the stress. She glanced at her watch to see if she had time before dinner to go to her bedroom, close the door, draw the blinds, and lie down. Maybe if she took a nap, she could reduce this headache before it became a migraine.

Then Nancy thought about an upcoming vacation with her family. She realized that if she was already struggling with a headache like this before the vacation even started, there was no way she could handle the car ride, the hotel, and the activities of a long weekend with her family. She decided right then that if she was going to go, she would drive herself, and it would be for just one day. Of course, that all depended on how she felt the morning everyone was getting ready to leave.

AVOIDANCE AND CONTROL

As Nancy struggled with the tension between managing her pain and going with her family on a short vacation, she felt none of her actions came from choices she consciously made. She managed her pain automatically, without thinking. If you were to ask her why she took the medication, went to lay down, opted out of committing to a family weekend, and controlled how she traveled, she most likely would say, "That is just how I manage pain. What else is there to do?"

We only have a sense of choice when we see there are two or more paths in front of us. If we only see one path, there is no sense of choice. Often, the things we do to manage our discomfort are done when we are on automatic pilot. We manage discomfort in ways that we have learned from our culture, from our family, and from figuring things out on our own through trial and error. The essence of our methods to handle discomfort is summed up by two words: avoidance and control.

When Nancy took her medication, went into a dark room and rested, opted out of activities, and controlled her circumstances, she was able to reduce her distress. She did not realize all of these strategies could be a trap. Once the distress-reducing effects of avoidance and control were over, she was right back where she started—with the same distress. We can also add to our distress with the type of control and avoidance strategies we use. Many of the most powerful distractions and pain reducers make our lives worse. Gambling, alcohol, caffeine, tobacco, food, sugar, drugs, inactivity, sleeping, and self-harm can make an already difficult life worse. Our solutions to our problems become yet one more problem in our lives.

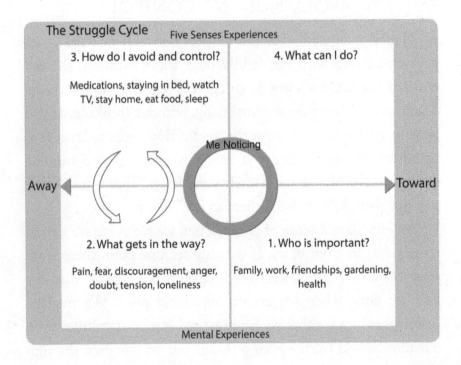

WHAT WE NOTICE

When we are stuck in the trap of experiencing distress and finding short-term relief through avoidance and control strategies, we are in a constant cycle of tension and relief. This cycle is called the *struggle cycle*. What we notice and pay attention to only includes our problems, pain, and methods to reduce distress.

Picture that center circle, which represents what we notice in the Matrix diagram, shifting over to the left side of the diagram. All that we see from day to day is our struggle with tension and short-term relief. The good things in life that bring real satisfaction seem remote and distant when we are trapped in the struggle cycle. Life does not feel vital or rich. The sense that we are living meaningful lives is gone, and we are left merely existing hour to hour, day to day. The struggle cycle is all that we can see when our spotlight of attention is only focused on what is getting in our way and what we can do to avoid and control our distress and discomfort.

WHAT WE CAN DO

Our attention gets stuck on the left side of the Matrix because of one fatal flaw in our thinking. We have a false belief that we would spend time and energy doing what is important to us as soon as we get rid of our distress and discomfort. We believe that the barriers to change are all those things that are getting in our way. Because of this false belief, we put all our attention and energy into getting rid of the distress and discomfort, which only makes the struggle cycle spin faster. Time keeps moving forward, but our lives never change—we stay stuck waiting to get rid of pain before we change direction.

Paying attention is an alternative to the struggle cycle. Noticing what is happening allows us to stand back from all that is going on and to see it from a distance. When we can see what is happening, we have the ability to make a choice to go in a different direction. When we do not notice what is happening and stay on autopilot, constantly reacting to life events, we remain stuck. In the following chapters, we will look at how to move from stuck to moving forward by increasing our awareness of our experiences from moment to moment.

18

• • •

DECIDING WHAT IS IMPORTANT

David was motivated to get better and was committed to putting in the work to get his life back. Due to his injury and the problems resulting from his multiple surgeries, he was left with chronic pain that became worse each month. It was hard for him to see his life going in the direction it was going. He tried his best to ignore his discouragement by doing projects around the house, but being a handyman at home does not pay the bills. David felt ashamed he could not provide for his wife. He was angry about what happened, angry at himself, and angry at life. David did not realize he was depressed.

Depression was not a concept that David understood well. He was pretty sure that people with depression just lay in bed all day feeling sorry for themselves. David thought old people and weak people got depressed, not him. He was physically and mentally strong. Before the accident, he saw himself as a self-made man. He worked hard, saved his money, did not complain, rarely worried, and slept well at night. But now things were different. He really did not know what to think of himself. He did not want to be around his old friends. They tried to stop by to see him, but he was less than welcoming. If he was invited to play cards or watch a sports game on TV, he would turn down the invitation. It was just too hard for him to predict what his pain would be like if he was trapped for hours socializing at someone's home.

David thought his poor sleep was related to pain, but when he began to talk about the problem with the psychologist, he realized that his mind did not let him sleep. He could not stop thinking about his future, the accident, the results of surgeries, and his wife. He would wake up at night after upsetting dreams and be chilled by cold sweats. One recurring dream was that his wife would leave him, and he would lose his home. When the psychologist asked him if he had talked about his stress and worry with his wife, the answer was no. He did not talk to her or anyone else about those issues. He felt they were his burden to carry, and he did not want to make things worse for anyone else. His physical problems were enough for his wife to face, he thought; she did not need to hear him complain about worrisome thoughts.

WHAT IS IMPORTANT

David expected the psychologist to give him a lecture on needing to open up to his wife or remind him that he needed to stop thinking such negative thoughts. But she didn't, which seemed strange to David. What was stranger still was when she asked him about what was important to him. Using the ACT Matrix diagram, she explained that what makes life meaningful and good are the people, ideas, beliefs, and values that are important to us. She suggested that as people pursue what is important to them without trying to change everything that is wrong, they are actually able to manage pain more effectively.[(1.)] She wondered how much time and energy David spent moving in step with his values.

Not only was David unsure about how much effort he put toward what was important to him, he had never thought about what was important to him, besides the fact that he loved his wife and extended family. To help David think about what was important, the psychologist asked him what kind of person he wanted to be when he was at work. His immediate response was that he wanted to be the guy that gets the job done. Then the psychologist followed up, "What was it about getting the job done that was so meaningful to you?"

David could feel the emotion well up in his chest as his eyes started to water. He replied, "I want to be a person that others can count on. I want to be a man who is respected. I want to be faithful and reliable because that is what it takes to make things work and make things better."

After a moment of silence, David explained that he had not realized until now what he really missed about his work. Yes, he missed not having a paycheck, but what he really missed was being the kind of person that made his workplace better. He encouraged others in the workplace and set a good example for the younger workers to follow. He liked being asked questions and giving advice that helped people work safely and efficiently. He loved that the leaders at his job all counted on him, looked up to him, and asked his input and advice about what was happening on the work floor. But now, all that was gone.

The psychologist had been writing some notes while David talked and showed him a list of words he had used: family, reliable, encouraging, helpful, dependable, kind, faithful, respect, mentor, and leader. She explained that these words were values and qualities that made his life meaningful and satisfying. David could not disagree. She then wanted David to think about if he was putting time and energy into living out his values now.

David thought for a moment and realized that even though he was not at work, there were still ways that he could still be the kind of person that was important to him. He could still show the same good character in his interactions with his family and friends. But looking at how he actually lived his life at home, he had to admit that he was not anything like the person that he wanted to be. He had emotionally walled off his wife, distanced himself from his extended family, and spent his evenings drinking beer, watching mindless things on TV, and ignoring his friends. Even though he kept himself busy during the day, the whole purpose of the different home projects was to distract himself from his pain.

DEFINING WHAT IS IMPORTANT

The psychologist gave David a home assignment. He was to look at five areas of his life and write out what kind of values he had in each area. These five areas included his relationships, work, leisure, learning, and health. There were other important areas that could be explored, but the psychologist knew that people often get overwhelmed with this exercise and are better off focusing on just a few key areas before adding others.

David was told to look at each of the five areas and write down some keywords, phrases, or sentences that described the person he wanted to be and the values he wanted to live out. Here are some questions that helped David think through each of these areas of his life.

- Relationships: What sort of brother, son, uncle, and husband do you want to be? What sort of relationships would you like to build? How would you interact with others if you were the "ideal you" in these relationships? How would you interact with your partner if you were the "ideal you" in that relationship? If you could be the best friend possible, how would you behave toward your friends?

- Work: What kind of contribution do you want to make in the world? What do you want to improve? What problems do you want to address with your abilities and talents? What kind of worker would you like to be? If you were living up to your own ideal standards, what personal qualities would you bring to your work? What sort of work relations would you like to build?

- Learning: What do you want to develop in yourself? What new skills would you like to learn? What knowledge would you like to gain?

- Leisure: What kind of activities help you become refreshed and energized? What sort of hobbies, sports, or leisure activities do you enjoy? What would you like to accomplish with leisure and refreshment?

- Health: Why is it important for you to look after your health? How do you want to look after your health with regard to sleep, diet, and exercise? What kind of habits do you want to develop to maintain your strength, flexibility, and cardiovascular system?

David was like many other motivated patients that the psychologist had seen before. When David saw the list of five areas of his life, he started listing the things he wanted to accomplish in each area. He wanted to improve his marriage, spend more time with his friends, start reading some good books, and get rid of his pain, at least for starters. Each of the items on David's list turned out to be a goal, not a value or quality he wanted to have in himself. Before he went further, he needed to learn about the difference between goals and values.

GOALS AND VALUES

David soon learned that a goal is something that can be checked off a list once it is accomplished. Goals are excellent to have, but they need to be linked to values. Values orient us; they are like a compass that points the way forward. We can value learning, but we will never learn everything. Goals for learning might be to read a book, take a class, or get a college degree. Once the goal is completed, we are done with the goal, but we can still live according to our values for the rest of our lives. Values help keep us on track to be the kind of person we want to become.

David had never really thought about his values before. But as he began to define the kind of husband, friend, sibling, son, worker, lifelong learner, and (eventually) father he wanted to become, he noticed that something was changing with his mood. By just talking about what was important to him, he began to feel better emotionally. He smiled when he was talking about someday having children. He thought back to the hobbies he used to enjoy and the way he spent time with friends. It was also becoming clear that he was not putting much energy and time into what was important to him at all. His efforts were focused on trying to control pain and distract himself from thinking about it. He wondered what he was supposed to do to make a shift toward living out his values.

He started creating a list of qualities and values that were important to him in each of the five areas. It did not matter if he was currently living them out or had never lived out the values or qualities in the past. The only criterion was that the personal qualities and values were important enough to him that he wanted to develop them and live them out. It was also important that he avoid listing values and qualities that were important to someone else. For example, his wife might want him to love classical music, but if this was not important to David, then it should not be on his list. When he completed his list, he was asked to sit down with his wife and talk about what was important to him. The goal of doing this was not to get her approval about his list, but to ask for feedback about what she saw as being important in his life. Sometimes other people who know us well can see what our values and qualities are more easily than we can see them ourselves.

SHORT-TERM GOALS

After David completed the values identification assignment, he was given a new task for the following week. For each of the values and qualities that David had listed in the values exercise, he needed to come up with some short-term and long-term goals. If healthy eating was an important value for David, a long-term goal could be to lose forty pounds. Two short-term goals for this week could be to drink eight eight-ounce glasses of water and eat three healthy meals daily. He could start doing both of these goals right now without needing any special extra resources or involvement from others.

David did indeed adopt these goals, which were right on target, but some of his first attempts at creating goals needed some help. The psychologist pointed out that David had selected several "dead man's goals." A dead man's goal is something that a dead person can do better than we can. David's initial goals were to avoid drinking soda and to stop smoking. Both of these goals a dead person can accomplish easily.

A goal that helps us move forward is something that we actively do, not something we avoid doing. Not drinking carbonated soft drinks is an excellent decision to make, but for healthy fluid intake to work as a goal, we need to find a replacement for the soft drinks. David's replacement for drinking soft drinks was to drink at least eight eight-ounce glasses of water per day. He would benefit from drinking even more, but since he hardly drank any water now, this was a good starting goal.

MAKING CHANGE HAPPEN

David completed his list of goals for each of the values and qualities he identified. His next assignment was simple—complete at least three goals each day and then write down the goals that he accomplished. It took a few days of doing this for David to realize what was happening as he focused on completing goals and living out his values. The first change he noticed was what he thought about in the morning. As he began his day, he looked over his list of values and goals and started to think through what he was going to accomplish that day. He had already started the habit of working on physical therapy and occupational therapy goals each day, but thinking about what was specifically important to him was new. Before this new habit started, he usually began the day with a sense of dread. Most mornings, he would try to figure out what plans he would need to cancel, activities he should probably avoid, and how his plans were going to end up being a problem and increase his pain.

Besides the change in how his mornings started, David also noticed a shift in how others around him interacted with him. As he intentionally worked on how he talked with his wife, asking her questions and talking about her day, it didn't take long for the atmosphere in their home to change. His wife, parents, and other relatives were no longer trying to stay out of David's way. They were no longer feeling anxious about trying to help with everything he did; David was no longer displaying his typical pain behavior as he got things done at home. David consciously worked at keeping his frustration and irritation out of sight. He started keeping his voice calm as he responded to questions. He wanted the way he communicated with his family to be consistent with one of his core values—make things better, not worse. As David focused on being the kind of person he wanted to be, the following pain behaviors naturally and gradually disappeared:

- Sighing when he sat down.
- Groaning when he got out of a chair, stood, and walked.
- Walking with a significant limp.
- Standing with his posture bent forward.
- Holding on to the wall as he walked.
- Using his cane.
- Wearing a back brace.
- Sleeping in the recliner, both day and night.
- Grimacing as he bent over, twisted, or lifted something.

FLARE-UPS

Just when David thought he was making progress, all of a sudden it was like he was back at square one. David's sister and her family had come to visit for a weekend, something that had not happened since his accident. About midway through the visit, David's back seized up, taking his breath away. Pain shot across his back, around to the front of his chest, and then down the back of both legs. He thought he was re-experiencing his original injury all over again. He was not sure what happened to cause the sudden increase in pain, which he tried to cover up as long as he could, but he eventually asked his wife to help get him to their bedroom so he could rest in bed.

The whole atmosphere in the home quickly changed when his pain flared up. David's sister was visibly upset, and she insisted they get David to a hospital. In an effort to calm his sister down, David tried to get out of bed, lost all the strength in his legs, and fell against the dresser, cutting open his forehead. David and his wife were able to keep the sister from calling 911, but in the end, they agreed to drive him to the emergency department to have his cut examined. At the hospital, David told his story of chronic pain and, to his surprise, was offered an injection of a muscle relaxer and prescription of an opioid to take home. David only agreed to take the muscle relaxer, in part to please his sister, who insisted he receive "real" medical treatment. David's forehead was fine and only needed cleaning up.

After his sister left town, David felt the trip to the hospital and taking the muscle relaxer was a huge step backward. He had tried so hard to make progress, and now he was back where he started. Beating himself up for not handling things better came easy to him; he had been doing this for years anytime he failed himself.

When David got back to see his physical therapist and psychologist the next week, he was already feeling much better but still did not know why his pain became so intense. When his pain flared up, so did the discouragement, doubt, frustration, and anxiety. The whole episode made David and his wife wonder if it was ever going to get better. David went back to being fearful of the future, distracting himself with mindless activities, being guarded and fearful of movement, and struggling with depression. He started looking on the internet for new medical procedures for back pain, including surgeries. He thought he would never consider surgery again, but part of him still held out hope for a magic bullet so he could get his old life back.

The physical therapist and psychologist both assured David that he was still on track for recovery and that flare-ups might happen. The pathways for chronic pain in the brain can get suddenly activated; it is hard to predict what set of circumstances can trigger those pathways. The way forward when flare-ups occur, they reminded him, was always the same—David needed to continue working on the things that got in the way of him moving toward his values and goals. The psychologist suggested that the pain flare-up provided a good opportunity to look at what thoughts, emotions, and sensations were getting David's attention and how the ways he wrestled with those issues possibly made his pain worse. That sounded good to David. We will see what he worked on in the next chapter.

19

• • •

GETTING HOOKED BY DIFFICULTY

Defining values and creating goals were exactly the kind of exercises David enjoyed. He saw himself as a man of action and loved the sense of accomplishment that came with a job well done. What he did not realize was sometimes it takes more than just determination to move toward what is important and overcome problems. Many things can get in our way as we take action, pursue goals, and seek to become the kind of person we know we can become. For David, self-doubt was now getting in his way of moving forward. He was struggling with his flare-up and recent emergency room visit. He wondered if all the progress he had made was for nothing. His mind was telling him he would never be pain-free, and if he could not be pain-free, what was the point of trying rehabilitation? David's problem went deeper than his flare-up or doubt, however. He needed to learn how his mind's method of problem-solving was a barrier to pursuing the life he wanted.

After the flare-up, David noticed that his pain levels were not dropping back to the level they had been in the past few weeks. He was proud of the progress he had made, but this new level of pain reminded him of the pain levels he had when the rehabilitation program started. Although he did not admit this to his wife or rehabilitation team, he was afraid. He was once again spending time awake at night wondering what he was doing wrong, how he could try harder, and what he needed to do to get rid of this pain once and for all.

THE PAIN-FREE TRAP

David did not look like himself when he arrived at the psychologist's office for his appointment. He was quieter than usual and looked stressed and unrested. Wanting to find out what was happening with David, the psychologist asked how he had been since the flare-up and emergency room visit. As David explained the details of the past few days, he used the phrase "pain-free life" several times. He said, "When this pain program started, I thought I was going to get back to my old self, 100 percent healthy and living a pain-free life again." The psychologist gave him some time to share his frustration and then suggested that David take a look at how his mind was working. Maybe how his mind was trying to solve his problems was a problem in itself.

The psychologist suggested that David do a small experiment and think of a time when he had done something of which he was ashamed. It only took a second for David to recall being ten years old and pressured by a friend to steal candy from a store. The moment David walked out of the store with the stolen goods, his father was walking into the store and saw the look of fear on David's face. David loved his dad, and the look of sadness and disappointment on his father's face was etched into his mind forever. David immediately walked back into the store and confessed his crime. The sting of that event had stayed with David all these years.

As David privately reflected on this memory, the psychologist asked David to banish the memory from existence. David was confused. How in the world was he supposed to get rid of a memory? Nevertheless, he tried to follow her suggestion. It seemed the more he tried to get rid of the thought, the more the memory and all the emotions associated with it came to the surface.

The psychologist then suggested that David try one more experiment. She asked him to think of a picture of a bright yellow Eiffel Tower in Paris—and then forget about it. David laughed as he tried his best to suppress the thought of a yellow Eiffel Tower, but the psychologist had made her point clear— what we do not want is what we end up getting. She explained that the mind is always trying to solve problems, but the method the mind uses to solve problems can create even more problems. She outlined on her notepad a cycle that occurs when difficult thoughts, experiences, memories, sensations, feelings, and images show up in our minds. She used David's recent flare-up as an example.

THE PAIN-FREE TRAP CYCLE

1. Unwanted Thoughts: First, a difficult thought shows up, such as, "I am a person with chronic pain, and I need to be pain-free to have a happy life." For David, the belief (also referred to as "a rule" in ACT therapy) that he needed to be pain-free in order to be happy was very strong. The thought hooked him.

2. Getting Hooked: The mind buys into these thoughts and regards them as true and valid. When we view our inner experiences as true and valid, we become fused with them. Fusion occurs when we get hooked by our thoughts, sensations, and emotions, which then carry us along in the direction they are going. David was carried along by his chronic pain thoughts because he assumed the thoughts were true.

3. Increased Distress: When we are hooked by a negative, difficult inner experience, we feel distressed and unhappy. The word machine inside our brain begins to tell a story, "I am so unlucky to be a chronic pain sufferer. I will never be able to be happy again. This makes me sad and discouraged." David's anxiety at night and irritation in the day were proof that he was distressed when he was hooked by such thoughts.

4. Avoidance and Control: We work hard at either getting rid of our discomfort or trying to avoid or suppress thoughts, emotions, memories, sensations, and images. In David's case, he tried to bury himself in projects, avoid thinking deeply, drink alcohol, and watch mindless TV to avoid and control unwanted thoughts.

5. Increased Tension: Whatever avoidance and control method we choose to use, we end up with even more tension because of the wrestling match between our good thoughts and our bad thoughts. As David increased his battle with unwanted thoughts, feelings, and sensations, his stress level started to rise, and the pain he experienced increased.

6. More Avoidance and Control: We might have some temporary relief, but once the distractions and methods of control and avoidance are over, we are back to where we started,

struggling with difficult experiences. For David, even when he could spend a whole day occupied with activity and an entire evening distracted by TV and alcohol, he still had to wake up the next morning with the same heavy weight on his mind from the day before: "I am a person with chronic pain. If I cannot become pain-free, I will never be happy." Along with those thoughts were also a large number of rules that his mind generated—rules like avoiding certain places, activities, and people to protect himself from pain, and rules for getting temporary pain relief by taking strong medication like muscle relaxers and sleeping in the reclining chair. When we get hooked by difficult thoughts, feelings, memories, and sensations, we also get hooked by all the rules that show up with difficult experiences.

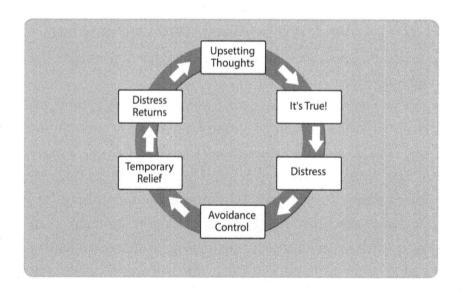

UNHOOKING FROM DIFFICULT EXPERIENCES

After using the Matrix to explain the struggle cycle that David was caught in, the psychologist pointed out how pointless it was for David to avoid, suppress, and control what happened in his mind. His painful memory from the past would always be with him. If he tried to get rid of the image of a bright yellow Eiffel Tower, it only appeared more often in his mind. What the psychologist suggested as an alternative to wrestling with unwanted experiences was to accept them and learn how to get unhooked by them.

We are not our thoughts. This concept is central to learning how to get unhooked. In some areas of your inner mental life, you already know that you are not your thoughts. You probably have had weird thoughts about yourself, other people, or the future. These weird thoughts occasionally show up, and you say to yourself, "Wow, that was weird. Where did that thought come from?" Everyone has strange thoughts and images that randomly occur. No big deal.

What you might not know is that you can look at thoughts, like "I will never be happy because I am a person with chronic pain," and do the same thing that you do with your strange, random thoughts. You can remind yourself that you are not your thoughts. In fact, it is helpful to look at your brain as a giant word-machine. The brain is constantly producing language, making connections, predicting, judging, evaluating, labeling, and creating stories about who you are and where your life is headed. That is the job of your brain.

THANKS, MIND!

To begin becoming unhooked, a good skill to practice is to simply thank your brain for all that work that it is doing trying to make sense of things. When a difficult thought shows up (e.g., "I am always going to have chronic pain, and that means my life is over."), you can say, "Thank you, mind, for trying to warn me and tell me who I am." The thought that you have chronic pain and that your life is over is not a bad thought. We do not need to replace it with a good thought. Unhooking from difficult thoughts happens when we stand back, notice the thought, and recognize that it is just a thought. After we notice the thought, we can be polite and thank our mind for sending it our way. By doing this, we are telling our brain not to treat these difficult thoughts as true or as a threat. If we react with fear and anxiety to difficult thoughts, we tell our brain that there is a serious threat.

FRONT-PAGE NEWS

Another simple unhooking strategy is to realize that your mind is a story-creating machine, not just a word-producing machine. Your mind is constantly trying to figure out what happened in the past, who you are now, and the direction your life is heading. When a person has chronic pain, the mind will create a very clear image of that person's life moving forward as one that is filled with pain, limitations, and loss.

We can unhook from the storytelling powers of the mind by realizing that our mind is like any modern news media outlet that wants us to stay on their station, website, and channel.[1.] News outlets are constantly promoting the next story that we cannot live without knowing about. Most people look at news outlets now and say, "Yeah, right! I think I can live without knowing what that actress ate for breakfast yesterday. Thanks anyway."

To practice this unhooking skill, picture yourself going through the checkout aisle at a large grocery store. On both sides of you are racks of candy and tabloid newspapers. On the cover of one newspapers is the headline, "Martians are secretly living in New York City." Then picture a headline about you and your life right next to the lead story about Martians. The headline reads, "You will always have chronic pain and never be happy."

Notice how your mind reacts to these two headlines. You do not say to yourself, "If that newspaper says there are Martians living in New York City, then I guess it is true." No, we don't say that at all. It does not matter that the news headline is in print or that millions of people buy the tabloid magazine. We know that the newspaper just wants us to get hooked by the story. Our minds are the same way. The mind wants our attention and wants us to listen in and believe the stories that it generates. We need to develop the skill of just looking at these stories as attention-getting devices that the mind is using, but not view them as true or useful.

ACCEPTANCE

In very large printed letters, the psychologist wrote one of David's recent thoughts on her notepad. It read, "I am a person with chronic pain, and I need to be pain-free to be happy." She then asked David to take the notepad and place it a few inches in front of his eyes so that the notepad was all that he could see. She then asked him about what that experience of only seeing the notepad was like. David replied, "Well, this is all that I can notice now. I cannot see anything else." She also asked if he tried hard enough, could he go through the day with the notepad in front of his face. The only thing he would really notice would be the notepad and that terrible sentence, "I am a person with chronic pain, and I need to be pain-free to be happy."

David was a quick learner. He had to admit, yes, this was a good picture of what he was doing. He probably had some moments when he was making progress and his attention was on moving forward, but since the pain flare-up, all his attention was focused on getting rid of his pain and the fear that he never would be pain-free.

The psychologist suggested that David now hold the notepad at arm's length to see what that was like. As he did, he realized that he could still see the notepad and the message on it, but he could also see many other things. He felt more engaged with the psychologist and connected to the rest of the things in the room. When David was wrestling with his thoughts, his attention was only focused on what was getting in his way. As he wrestled with the yucky stuff in his way, the more difficult thoughts, emotions, and sensations he wanted to get rid of pushed back. But when he stopped pushing, avoiding, controlling, and focusing on the difficult thoughts and emotions, the struggle came to an end, and he could focus on other things, especially things that were important to him, like his family.

The psychologist described the process of letting go of the struggle as a step toward acceptance.[2.] Acceptance did not sound like a word that David liked to hear, especially in connection with chronic pain. Why would he want to accept pain? He wanted to get rid of it and be pain-free, not accept it!

To help David look at acceptance from a different perspective, the psychologist used the illustration of a person stuck in quicksand. There are very few places in the world were natural quicksand traps occur, but they do exist. If a person steps into quicksand, the natural instinct is to struggle. The more a person struggles, they create a vacuum beneath themselves and begin to sink further down. The only way to survive in quicksand is to stop struggling, lean back, and spread your arms and legs. Doing this goes against every instinct that we have, but science will tell us that the human body is buoyant and will float in water. Quicksand traps are made mostly of water. If we simply stay still and lean into the difficult experience of the quicksand, we can become less entangled and then free ourselves.

David could see himself struggling for his life, not just in the quicksand, but with all the negative thoughts, feelings, and sensations that kept coming up. He honestly had never thought of just accepting those difficult experiences. The psychologist explained that acceptance does not need to mean "I like this!" It simply means that we allow the difficult things in our lives to be there without trying to change them or avoid them. Another word that is often used for acceptance in ACT therapy is *willingness*. When we are willing, we move toward the difficulty we are experiencing with openness and curiosity. We don't just turn away from it.

The psychologist reminded David that acceptance was not the same as tolerance. When we tolerate a difficult person, we put up with them. But with willingness and acceptance, we look at every difficult experience we have as something we can explore, learn from, be open about, and allow in our lives. She then asked, "David, if you worked at accepting pain, what do you think would happen in your brain? How would your brain view your pain if you constantly said to yourself that it is okay that you have pain?" David replied, "I suppose my brain would wonder why it needs to be cranking out so much pain if I do not even think pain is a problem."

RECOVERY FROM DEPRESSION

A few days after discovering acceptance and working on specific goals, David had a new experience as he was lying in bed getting ready to fall asleep. He was actually looking forward to the next day. Ever since his accident, he had always dreaded what was to come. But not now.

The pain in his lower back and legs were still a part of his life, but he was now managing flare-ups with stretches and exercises. He was walking longer distances, which helped greatly in managing stress and improving his sleep. He was able to manage pain more easily with breathing exercises, progressive muscle relaxation, and acceptance. Before he drifted off to sleep, he thought about all the positive changes that had occurred recently in his life and was convinced his decision to stop waiting for his pain to go away and to start moving toward what was important was the key to his recovery. This decision to move forward and not get stuck avoiding and controlling pain also brought an end to his depression. The emotional weight he was feeling, the social isolation he experienced, the sleeplessness and darkness he felt about himself and his future were beginning to lift.

20

• • •

HOW TO GET UNSTUCK

Ever since her recent trip to the emergency room for her panic attack, Rachel mostly focused on her pain and fatigue. Her attention was hooked on her stress and anxiety, leaving her wondering if her anxiety was going to get out of control. The more Rachel wrestled with her anxiety and tried to control her pain, the more frustrated and stuck she felt. When she was at home, she managed both the pain and anxiety by lying in bed, closing the bedroom door, and telling her children they needed to do something on their own while she got some rest. This habit of spending time in bed went from a once- or twice-a-week occurrence to a daily habit when she arrived home from the office.

To get through her workday, she relied on chemical coping. Caffeine kept her awake, alert, and going to the bathroom, and medications helped to get her to sleep at night. The caffeine also increased her level of pain, which she did not realize until the psychologist told her. She used ibuprofen and acetaminophen constantly, unaware of the health risks involved in their daily use.

PAYING ATTENTION

Rachel completed the values inventory assignment early on in her pain rehab program. She knew what was important to her and could picture what kind of person she wanted to be, even in the middle of this difficult time of her life. Yet, she was convinced she had no time, energy, or physical strength to move toward what was important to her. All her energy was wrapped up in trying to control her pain and anxiety.

She looked at her blank copy of the ACT Matrix and began to wonder if what the psychologist had been talking about might be helpful to her. She was desperate to find a way to get her life back under her control; she hoped there was something in the Matrix that could help.

As she looked at the diagram, the circle in the center of the Matrix got her attention. She remembered that the circle symbolized a person paying attention to external experiences through the five senses as well as the internal, private experience of the mind. She realized that she was not at all aware of what was happening in some areas of her life. Her attention was hooked on the area labeled, "What gets in the way."

She got a pen out and started to write what got in her way: anxiety, pain, fear, worry, tightness in her chest, soreness, fear of not sleeping, fatigue, irritation, guilt, sadness, work stress, stiffness, brain fog, memories of her emotional and physical decline over the years, recent arguments with her husband, images of the sad expressions on her children's faces when she tells them once again she cannot play with them, and mental pictures of the ideal wife, loving mother, and successful businesswoman that she felt she would never become. Just writing

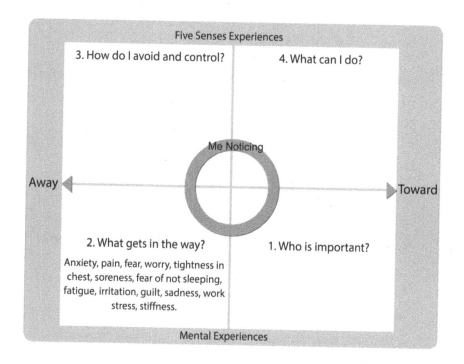

Five Senses Experiences

3. How do I avoid and control?

4. What can I do?

Me Noticing

Away ◄————————————————►Toward

2. What gets in the way?

Anxiety, pain, fear, worry, tightness in
chest, soreness, fear of not sleeping,
fatigue, irritation, guilt, sadness, work
stress, stiffness.

1. Who is important?

Mental Experiences

down what got in her way made her more depressed. She began
to wonder why she was doing this exercise.

The psychologist had suggested in one of their recent sessions that Rachel would benefit from noticing more about what
she did when difficult experiences showed up. He suggested
that it was often hard to notice what we do because our behavior
seems so natural to us, happening as if we are on autopilot.
Rachel wondered what could be so hard about noticing how she
coped with difficulty. After all, she really did not do very much
when pain showed up, besides take a few over-the-counter
medications and rest. She reasoned that, given her painful condition, most people would consider this a pretty normal coping
strategy. She got out the worksheet the psychologist had given
her on how to recognize avoidance and control strategies—
strategies we often use when we are on autopilot.

CONNECTING THE DOTS

The strategies that we use to reduce tension and avoid distress can be remembered by the acronym DOTS, which stands for the following: (1.)

- D—Distraction: We distract ourselves from difficult thoughts, feelings, and sensations by watching TV, shopping, playing video games, gambling, pursuing hobbies, reading, working, exercising, volunteering, helping, sleeping, cleaning, or using the internet.
- O—Opting Out: To manage our discomfort and distress, we can opt out, quit, avoid, or withdraw from people, places, activities, and situations when we are uncomfortable. Rather than going to a large grocery store that requires more walking, we opt out and go to a small convenience store nearby.
- T—Thinking and Talking: We try to analyze what is happening to us, or we talk about our struggles constantly. We can read information about our problem, consult with experts, worry, rehash the past, fantasize, think positive thoughts to overcome negative thoughts, problem-solve, and plan. We can spend a great deal of time wondering about what-ifs, if-only's, and why-me's. We can also blame ourselves, blame others, or blame our past.
- S—Substances and Self-harm: We can cope by using substances such as food, alcohol, cigarettes, caffeine, marijuana, over-the-counter medications, sleeping pills, sex, and prescription medication. We can also use self-harming activities, such as suicide attempts or reckless risk-taking.

Rachel remembered the psychologist explaining to her that distraction, opting out, thinking, talking, substances, and self-harm were powerful tools in reducing discomfort. We would not turn to these DOTS strategies if they were not effective at helping us feel less bad. Some of the strategies can even help us temporarily feel good, but they also have negative consequences that create more problems in our lives. Staying in bed feels good for a while, but it will result in a person becoming weak, stiff, and sore from the lack of activity and blood flow. Smoking and drinking alcohol also feel good in the short term but have long-term negative consequences. This made sense to Rachel, but she wondered how thinking and talking could be such a problem.

As Rachel looked at the list of thinking and talking strategies, she recognized that this was her core coping strategy. She was constantly trying to discern what was wrong, what she should do, and whom should she consult. She read all the latest articles and research on fibromyalgia. What she read often made her more upset. She talked about her pain and anxiety constantly with her husband, mother, sister, and girlfriends.

Upon recognizing that thinking and talking may be one of her strategies to control and avoid her distress, she immediately became defensive. She told herself, "What else am I supposed to do? I cannot just ignore my problems and stick my head in the sand!" That was when she remembered what the psychologist had mentioned about the thinking and talking strategies—they give a person a feeling that they are doing something, just like being in a rocking chair gives a person a feeling of being active. After twenty minutes in a rocking chair, a person is still in the same place they were when they started rocking. After a long day of using thinking and talking strategies, no real change has occurred. When Rachel's time spent thinking and talking were over, the struggles, tension, and distress she was avoiding came right back up to the surface.

THE STRUGGLE CYCLE

As Rachel began to look harder, she could see that she used strategies from all four categories. She distracted herself with TV, reading, and work. There were many activities, events, and places that she avoided. She used talking and thinking the most, which kept her awake throughout the night. She depended on prescribed medications, caffeine, over-the-counter medications, and sleeping pills to cope from day to day. All of these strategies had the very predictable short-term positive effect of reducing her tension and distress, but that was it.

When she looked at the Matrix, she could see that what got her attention was only the left side of the diagram. All she noticed was the cycle of experiencing anxiety, pain, and distress, and then working hard to control or avoid her discomfort. This is what her psychologist called the struggle cycle.[2.] The more she relied on the avoidance and control strategies, the faster the struggle cycle spun.

Now that she was recognizing this cycle in her life, she wondered what else she was supposed to do instead of just struggle. The psychologist explained the struggle cycle was fueled by a false belief, which states: "I will focus on what is important to me as soon as I get rid of all this stuff that is getting in my way first." Of course, we never get rid of all that gets in our way. To manage our tension, we keep on relying on strategies that make the struggle cycle spin faster, like distraction, opting out, talking and thinking, and substances or self-harm. In the end, all our attention stays on the left side of the Matrix, and the things that make life rich and rewarding become distant and remote. The values, character traits, and desires that make life rich and meaningful do not come into focus or get noticed.

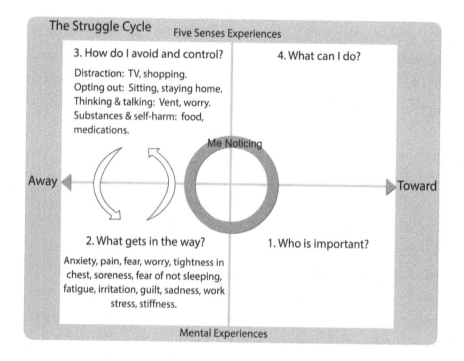

GETTING PRESENT

During her next psychology appointment, Rachel shared her discoveries about being stuck in the struggle cycle. She wanted to know what the alternatives were to the DOTS strategies. How was she supposed to jump off the merry-go-round that she was stuck on? To address her question, the psychologist asked Rachel if she would be willing to do an experiment.

The experiment involved Rachel taking a deep breath in through her nose and letting it out slowly with her mouth, focusing all her attention on her breath. After focusing all her attention on her breath for a few moments, she was asked to look around the room and notice five things that she could see. With that task completed, she then was asked to notice four different physical sensations anywhere on her body. She then needed to listen for and identify at least three different sounds, either nearby sounds or sounds further away. With her sense of smell, she was to identify at least two different smells. Finally, she was asked to notice the sense of taste in her mouth. At the end of the experiment, Rachel directed her attention back to her breath for a few moments. (To hear an audio version of this exercise, go to: PainRehabSource.com)

This simple exercise of noticing her environment with her five senses helped Rachel in an unexpected way. During the exercise, she was not focused on anxiety, pain, problems, or worries because her attention was in the present moment. The psychologist explained that focusing attention on noticing five-sense experiences does not allow the mind to go toward the past or the future. When we struggle, we are generally struggling with thoughts and feelings that are connected to the past or the future, not to the present moment.

He asked Rachel, "When you spend time reading, talking, thinking, and analyzing your problems, where is your mind? Is your focus in the present, the past, or the future?" She stated it was often in the future, wondering what will happen next. But her mind was also in the past, wondering why all this happened and what could she have done to stop the fibromyalgia and anxiety from developing. He then asked, "What does it cost you when you spend a lot of time with your attention directed toward the past or your attention directed at the future?" It took only a moment of reflection to know the answer—it cost her losing out on the present moment. It cost her missing out on life as it happened.

Rachel thought back to all the meals she had eaten with her family when she was physically sitting at the table, but her mind was trapped in the struggle cycle. Her children and husband often had to tap her arm and ask, "Are you listening to us?" As she tried to sleep, her mind would be replaying the events of the day and bracing herself for events yet to come the next day.

The psychologist took out the Matrix diagram and pointed to the lower-left corner. He explained that when all of our attention is on what is getting in our way, we actually lose contact with five-sense experiences and the important people in our lives. But something else happens when the focus of our attention is on what gets in our way. We can imagine past or future events so clearly that we have strong emotional and physical responses to what we are imagining as if these events were actually happening in the present moment. This happens because we treat our thoughts as if they are true and valid.

Rachel could see how her problem-solving mind was getting in her way of how she wanted to live life. Every weekend, she wondered if she should go to church with her family. The day before the church service, she would picture herself sitting in the church in pain, unable to use any of her favorite distraction strategies, suffering for ninety minutes, and then having a pain flare-up for the rest of the day. She wondered, "If I am always picturing the worst, is my body just bracing for the problems before they even happen?" She knew the answer before she asked the question—yes, her body was anticipating a threat and preparing her for the threat by producing pain, even before anything happened.

LEAVES ON A STREAM

The psychologist encouraged Rachel to practice noticing her thoughts, feelings, sensations, memories, and images as if they were just cars passing by as she stood on the edge of a road. As an alternative, he suggested that she could picture the thoughts and mental events as individual clouds passing through a wide-open blue sky or as leaves floating by on a stream. Rachel's task was to notice each event (thought, feeling, sensation, memory, or image) as it occurred and notice the mental events coming to her awareness, passing in front of her, and then moving on like a car passing her on the road, a cloud traveling through the open sky, or a leaf on a river. The individual cars or clouds or leaves do not represent who she is as a person. They are just single events that show up, pass through her life, and move on, only to be replaced by something else in the next moment. (To hear an audio version of this exercise, go to my website: PainRehabSource.com)

As Rachel practiced this in the office during the psychology session and then at home, it became clear that it was very hard for her to bring her attention to the present moment and stay there. She was getting carried away on every other leaf that floated down the stream.

EXPANSION

As Rachel practiced staying present and noticing her thoughts, feelings, sensations, memories, and images, she began to catch herself using her avoidance and control strategies to temporarily reduce her discomfort. Paying attention to what was happening helped her to start connecting the DOTS. With repeated effort and practice, she noticed the entire struggle cycle instead of being stuck in it. Once she began to notice what she was doing, she suddenly experienced the sense of having a choice. She could either move away from what was uncomfortable and difficult, or she could pay attention to what is important to her and move toward her values. If she moved toward her values, she could express the kind of behavior and character that she considered important. She wanted to be loving, engaged, interested in others, present, patient, courageous, hopeful, and helpful.

Paying attention to what was happening in her mind, in her five-sense experiences, and to the choices she was making, gave her a sense of hope. Maybe she was not going to stay stuck in the struggle cycle forever, especially if she could learn better ways to manage her physical pain. She benefited from the stretching, strength training, and cardio exercises she was learning from physical and occupational therapy, but she could not use those strategies if she was sitting in a meeting for two hours.

The psychologist presented a way of looking at pain that she could experiment with. He called this the *expansion mind-set*, and it involves making room for difficult things in our lives.[3.] This way of looking at pain involves three processes:

1. Observe: Notice where the pain is located. Is it still or moving? Is it big or small? Are the sensations strong or weak? Where is the center of the pain, and where is the edge? The goal of observing is simply to be curious and

open to what is there without judging, evaluating, or controlling.

2. Breathe: Visualize where the pain is located and then slowly breathe in and imagine that the air is moving directly to and around the pain. Picture the air penetrating and surrounding the pain.

3. Acceptance: Allow the difficult sensations to be present, even if you do not like them. Picture yourself making space for the pain. Create a small room filled with the warm air that surrounds your pain. Any time your mind tries to resist accepting the discomfort, just say, "Thank you, mind!"

Several days had gone by since that last psychology session. Rachel was consistently working on paying attention, staying present, and making room for her painful sensations, emotions, and thoughts. One night, both she and her husband were busy with the children's bedtime routine, when she overheard her older daughter talking to her husband. Her husband was kneeling next to the bed saying goodnight, and her daughter softly said, "I am so glad Mom is back." Her husband asked what she meant. The daughter replied, "I don't have to tell Mom something three times now. She hears me the first time. Mom is not grumpy when she tries to help me with homework, and she smiles now."

Rachel cried herself to sleep that night. She was not upset at herself, depressed about her life, or despondent about her future. The tears flowed because she was relieved that she was no longer stuck in the struggle cycle and that someone else had noticed. The people she loved the most could tell she was different. The people she loved the most could sense she loved them.

21

• • •

MOVING FORWARD

Rachel noticed changes in life as she began to pay attention to the choices she made and to what was going on around her and inside her mind. She was choosing to spend less time in bed, going out with her husband for dinner with friends, and relying less on her medications and caffeine to get through her workday. Her husband and children noticed the differences and told her that she sounded and looked better. She liked how she was functioning, but she could not shake the sense of guilt and pressure she felt each day.

The guilt and pressure Rachel experienced showed up at work, at home, while running errands, and even when she was taking ten minutes to do a simple breathing exercise. She began to talk about her feelings of guilt one night with a girlfriend who stopped by for a visit. What was not obvious to Rachel about her struggle with guilt and pressure was obvious to her lifelong friend.

Her girlfriend had no trouble telling Rachel what seemed obvious. She explained, "Rachel, you have always done well at school and sports. You push yourself. That is a great quality about who you are, and it helps you to be successful. But as long as I have known you, you've measured your worth as a person by what you accomplish. If you do not have the outcome you want at home or at work, or if you do not feel you have control, you feel like a failure. It is no wonder you feel guilty all the time. By measuring yourself by what you accomplish, you probably think you are always coming up short. Even though you look successful to most people, I know that you often feel worthless and get angry at yourself when you can't meet your own expectations. This way of living has to be hard on you emotionally and physically."

THE EULOGY

As they talked, Rachel wondered if her girlfriend was right. She did measure herself and was always coming up short, feeling inadequate and angry. Was the measure she had for her sense of worth wrong? What was she supposed to replace it with? After her girlfriend left, Rachel looked through her notes and home assignments from the psychologist. There was a short exercise on writing a eulogy for herself that she was supposed to work on. She was to picture herself at her own funeral with all her friends and family standing around her graveside waiting to hear the eulogy summarizing the highlights of her life.[1.] The home assignment was for her to write out what she would like to have done with her life and the legacy she would want to leave to her children and grandchildren.

As Rachel worked on this exercise, it only took her a few minutes to make the connection between the pressure she felt, her guilt, and what was missing in her life. As she wrote her eulogy, she never mentioned her success at work, getting approval from others, the sales goals for her division, recognition from professional marketing organizations, her year-end productivity bonus, the orderliness of her house, or having perfect children or an ideal marriage. None of these things are what she wanted to be remembered for, but somehow, she had selected all of these goals as a measuring rod of what she thought was supposed to be a good life. When she completed the exercise, she knew she had to find a different direction for her life and develop a better standard to measure how well she was doing.

THE MOVIE

In order to encourage Rachel to think creatively about where to steer her life, the psychologist asked Rachel to pretend a movie was going to depict her life as a pain-free individual. She was supposed to imagine she had miraculously become totally pain-free and could do whatever she wanted in life. For this imaginary exercise, her job was to sit down with the actress who would portray her and describe how she would talk, spend her time, react to people, handle frustrations, spend time with her children, interact with her husband, dress, and sound as an individual who experienced a miracle cure.

The psychologist took out the Matrix diagram once again and pointed to the upper-right corner labeled, "What I can do." Thinking of what she would do if she were not held back by pain helped Rachel focus on what she could do to move forward—in a direction that was important to her. Rachel listed the friends she wanted to spend time with, memories she wanted to make with her husband and children, friendships she wanted to renew, ways she could help and support her parents, attitudes she wanted to have when she was at work, volunteering she wanted to do in the community, and qualities she wanted to have to make a positive impact on others.

Looking at her list, Rachel felt a mixture of excitement and despair. On the one hand, it was like a roadmap pointing in the direction she wanted to go with her life. On the other hand, she still felt the weight of her anxiety, pain, guilt, and pressure. The miracle cure wasn't real, and there was no actress who was going to portray her marvelous new life. In the real world, she had things that still got in her way. What was she supposed to do about all the things holding her back?

THE WAGON

As Rachel discussed her inner conflict and tension with the psychologist, he asked her to look at the list she created and identify actions she could engage in right now, even in the condition she was in with her pain, anxiety, pressure, and guilt. That was not hard to do for Rachel. There were several things she could do, in part because there were so many simple activities and behaviors on her list. She could call an old friend, make crafts with her children, be patient, spend time with her husband, listen attentively, and build better relationships at work. She did not have to wait for something to change with her pain or anxiety to do these simple things.

The psychologist asked Rachel to picture all the thoughts, sensations, memories, images, emotions, and self-concepts that got in her way as toys sitting in a red children's wagon. Rachel was asked to give up on trying to get rid of everything in that wagon and instead pick up the handle and pull the wagon and all things in it with her as she moved toward what is important to her.

Rachel recognized that she had already started to do this, but moving forward with this wagon went against her wish to get rid of all her problems first. She felt pressure to make things right, fix problems, eliminate the mess, and make things look good. Dragging a wagon full of junk with her was not Rachel's idea of a good time. As she said this out loud, she could hear the response in her mind, "What other choice do you have?" None. There was no getting rid of it all or making things look perfect. She would have to move forward in the condition she was in now.

THE MONSTERS ON THE BUS

Choosing to move forward is not a one-time decision but a series of choices made at every moment. To help Rachel experience this concept, the psychologist introduced her to one of his favorite thought experiments: the monsters on the bus.[2] He asked her to picture being the driver of a large public bus. As she drove her bus route, she would pick up a variety of passengers and drop them off along the route at different bus stops. As the bus driver, Rachel kept to a specific route each day, and the passengers needed to stay on the route with her until their assigned stop.

Rachel was then asked to imagine that, one day, she started to pick up some undesirable passengers along her route—real monsters. When these frightening creatures got on the bus, they started making noise, upsetting Rachel and making her job miserable. Rachel decided she was going to throw them off the bus, but it did not work because the monsters far outnumbered her, so she could not catch or control them. She then decided to bring the bus back to the bus station. That is when things got worse.

As soon as Rachel started heading in that direction, the monsters started to threaten her, scare her, and jump around on the bus. They made all kinds of noise and demanded that she go in the opposite direction of her desired destination, the bus station. They did not care where she went as long as it was not to the bus station, and if she seemed to be heading that way, they'd threaten her again. The psychologist paused and had Rachel list the monsters in her life: pain, fear of pain, pain catastrophizing, the pressure to perform well, anxiety, feelings of inadequacy, memories of past failure, fatigue, and high expectations. All these issues stood in the way of the life she really wanted, just like the monsters on the bus.

The psychologist asked Rachel what happened when she listened to the monsters on the bus. "The truth is," started Rachel, "I end up listening to the monsters for days in a row, driving in circles, exhausted from fear. I do not let myself just go in the direction I want to go." The psychologist suggested that this nightmare could end if a new idea came to her mind.

He suggested, "What if the monsters are just ghosts? What if all they can do is threaten, yell, and scream? What if they cannot really touch you or stop you from doing things?" If this were true, Rachel could stop trying to throw the monsters off the bus and driving in circles. She could head directly where she wanted to go. The psychologist reminded her that the closer she got to the bus station, the louder she should expect the monsters to be. But if she just kept driving, she would eventually arrive safely at her desired destination.

THE STRUGGLE SWITCH

Rachel thought about the monsters-on-the-bus metaphor and how it applied to her own life. She really wanted to throw those monsters off her bus! They scared and threatened her. Her thoughts, emotions, sensations, memories, and self-concepts all had more influence over her life than she wanted. It was hard for her to accept that getting rid of all her yucky stuff was not a viable option.

Like most people at this point in their struggle to move forward, Rachel was waiting for something to happen to make change easier. But then she recognized this thought was a trap. Change was not going to be easy. So, she decided to go in a new direction. She would choose to move forward and do what was important to her and not wait to get rid of everything in her way. That was all she did—she made a choice to take committed action.

As Rachel started on this new way of living, she found that she had to continually make the same choice. She pictured her mind as having a "struggle switch" that was either turned on or off.[3.] If the struggle switch was turned on, she was choosing to wrestle with her monsters by trying to throw them off the bus. If the struggle switch was off, she was choosing to move forward with a busload of crazy monsters toward what was important to her, ignoring the option to struggle with the monsters. If the struggle switch was on, that was her choice. She would fight with the monsters until she chose otherwise. When the struggle switch was off, that, too, was her choice. She came to the important realization that everything she did was a choice. Her choices helped her move either in a direction that was important to her or further away from what was important.

THE SATISFACTION CYCLE

Rachel was now taking steps to move toward what was important to her. What she discovered was that she was less aware of anxiety, fatigue, pain, and pressure. This did not make sense because she was not trying to get rid of her distress. In fact, she did not know why her old monsters were not as noisy and upsetting. The psychologist got the Matrix out for one last teaching point.

He drew arrows connecting the two areas on the right side of the Matrix, the upper-right section (What can I do?) and the

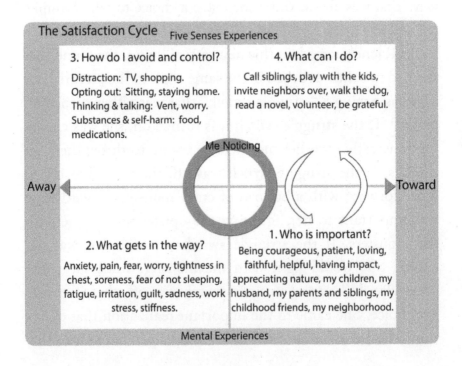

The Satisfaction Cycle   Five Senses Experiences

3. How do I avoid and control?

Distraction: TV, shopping.
Opting out: Sitting, staying home.
Thinking & talking: Vent, worry.
Substances & self-harm: food, medications.

4. What can I do?

Call siblings, play with the kids, invite neighbors over, walk the dog, read a novel, volunteer, be grateful.

Me Noticing

Away ← → Toward

2. What gets in the way?

Anxiety, pain, fear, worry, tightness in chest, soreness, fear of not sleeping, fatigue, irritation, guilt, sadness, work stress, stiffness.

1. Who is important?

Being courageous, patient, loving, faithful, helpful, having impact, appreciating nature, my children, my husband, my parents and siblings, my childhood friends, my neighborhood.

Mental Experiences

lower-right section (What is important?). He explained that Rachel had now engaged the satisfaction cycle. As her behavior, actions, and choices became in line with what she believed to be important, valuable, and worthwhile, Rachel enjoyed the sense of satisfaction that came from doing what she knew to be good. Rachel found it interesting that some of the items on her avoid-and-control list were also on her what-I-can-do? list. She realized that it was not really the activity itself that was good or bad. What mattered was the function it served—in other words, why she did it. What was important to her now was making sure that everything she did served her values. This made all the difference when it came to her sense of meaning, purpose, and satisfaction as she went about her day.

As Rachel spent time doing what was important to her, her brain produced endorphins that caused happy feelings. The endorphins traveled from her brain and down her spine, putting up gates that limited the information coming up about pain. In addition, as Rachel's focus shifted away from her pain and anxiety toward what was rewarding and satisfying, the sense of threat that her brain had about pain began to turn down. As the threat level lowered in her brain, so did the brain's pain output. Even though Rachel's decision to move forward was not a tricky attempt to get rid of her monsters and yucky feelings, in the end, her monsters were quieter and less significant in her life.

22

• • •

CONCLUSION

David, Rachel, and Nancy are normal people who struggle with change. Regardless of the improvement they experienced over the course of their treatments, they occasionally forgot what they learned. They forgot the amount of effort it took to keep stretching and exercising every day. Some days, they followed their usual approach of getting things done and forgetting to use their pacing strategies. They fell out of the habit of doing breathing exercises every morning and evening. When they were in the middle of a rehabilitation program, it was not hard to remember all their pain management principles because they were meeting regularly with a team that knew their progress, habits, and struggles. After the program, it was important for each of them to get the support and encouragement they needed to stay on track. Follow-up visits with their rehab support team and talking with others who successfully learned to manage pain were both key to ongoing progress.

Pain is a powerful motivator. The return of old pain, physical limitations, sleep loss, and stress reminds many pain patients that they need to go back to the basics of active pain management. Typically, even a person who has progressed well with their pain rehabilitation will have occasional relapses. The result of that rehabilitation, however, is a change in recovery time. When former pain rehabilitation patients experience increased pain, their recovery time is generally much shorter.

To guard against returning to old habits and passive ways of managing pain, it is important to know when problems will occur. For example, the healthcare system that pain patients need to navigate will promote standard pain management approaches that can leave a person with even more pain and medical problems. Friends and family who see someone struggle with pain want to help, not knowing that the help they offer can actually make things worse. To prepare for these and other challenges, we will review the five key principles of pain management covered in the three sections of this book. The truth is, we always need to keep reviewing what we learn because our memories are poor. Good reminders will keep us progressing toward better health.

Not everyone will rely on all five strategies when managing pain. You may have already found that some of these skills are more useful to you than others. Review these five principles often and let your accountability partners know the habits, attitudes, and mindset you are developing.

1. UNDERSTANDING THE BIG PICTURE

Everyone with chronic pain has at least two questions: "Why am I in so much pain?" and "Why won't the pain stop?" To answer these questions, we need to know something about the nervous system and how the brain responds to the information it receives from damaged areas of the body.

The nervous system specializes in detecting change and problems in the body. Specialized nerves gather information for the brain and provide the input the brain needs. When we have a disc that puts pressure on a nerve in our back, or when we have tissue damage from a torn muscle or ligament, the changes are picked up by specialized nerves and sent to the brain for processing. The nerves do not send pain information—they only send information that something has changed. It is the brain that needs to determine if the changes that have occurred deserve a pain signal.

When the brain attempts to explain what is happening, there can be problems with the conclusions it makes if it lacks all the information that it needs. The brain uses a scale to determine if it needs to produce pain or not. On one side of the scale is credible evidence for danger, and on the other side of the scale is credible evidence for safety. We call these two parts of the scale danger-in-me (DIM) and safety-in-me (SIM). When there is more evidence for danger than safety, pain will be produced.

When we experience pain, another protective system will be triggered in our bodies. Pain activates the stress alarm system, which triggers the fight-flight-freeze response. Because of our stress response, our muscles become tense, blood circulation changes, hormone and blood sugar levels change, and inflammation increases in many areas of the body. All of these changes can lead to increased pain levels. Many other life events and emotional issues, such as fear, stress, anxiety, anger, loneliness, and history of past trauma, can also influence how intensely we experience pain. Having this broad understanding of how pain works in the body is vital to understanding how pain management techniques impact the body.

2. CALMING

There are many different strategies that can help turn off the stress alarm system when it is triggered by pain. When we are in pain, our body becomes tense, and our breathing, heart rate, and blood pressure all increase. One skill that is more helpful than any other is diaphragmatic breathing, also called belly breathing. The basics of diaphragmatic breathing include breathing slowly in through the nose, out through the mouth, and focusing our attention on the gentle movement of the stomach as it moves with each breath. The stomach, not the chest, should move out with every inhale and in with every exhale.

To benefit from this breathing exercise, practice for ten minutes a day, twice a day. Once you have spent time practicing a breathing strategy, then it is time to use other calming techniques that help stimulate the release of calming hormones called endorphins. Some of these mindfulness strategies include the body scan or mindful awareness of the five senses.

3. ACCEPTANCE AND WILLINGNESS

Acceptance means making room in our life for something that is difficult. It is best understood as allowing something to be in our life without struggle, avoidance, or attempts to control it. Pain is made worse by our attempts to make it go away. We do not need to pretend we like pain, and we definitely do not want to try to convince ourselves that we are not in pain when we are.

The opposite of acceptance is to engage in a wrestling match with what we do not want in our life. The simple statement "If you are not willing to have it, you will" sums up the paradox of not accepting difficulty. The very thing we try to avoid is what we end up getting. If we try to get rid of anxiety, we get more anxiety. The same is true of pain.

When we learn to welcome and make room for the difficult experiences in our life, an important change takes place within our brain—acceptance interferes with our brain's ability to view pain as a terrible threat. We usually look at pain as a catastrophe. As a result, we have catastrophic thoughts about what will happen in the future, how much we will suffer, and picture our life in very dark terms. If you want to change the balance of the DIM and SIM scale in your brain, then acceptance can be a powerful tool to help your brain to stop viewing pain as a terrible threat.

4. BALANCING

There are two main elements of maintaining balance while living with chronic pain: pacing and boundaries. Pacing begins by learning how to be aware of your body and what you are doing when you are engaged in activities. If you are working around the house, learn to pay attention to how much energy you have and what your body is telling you. Your body will tell you when discomfort and tiredness are starting, but only if you are paying attention.

Pacing involves learning to be active and yet comfortable by staying in your discomfort zone for short periods of time. After ten to fifteen minutes of activity, take a short break. You might be sore or uncomfortable during that period of activity, or you may be completely comfortable. The goal is to avoid pushing too hard or going all the way through your discomfort zone up past your pain threshold. If you push yourself into your pain region, other problems occur. Once you are in pain, your brain will associate the activity you are doing with pain. Pacing, when done correctly, will help your brain relearn that movement and activity do not need to be associated with pain.

When you apply pacing correctly, you may find that you can be more active than you expected. This can usher in a new set of problems—learning to say no to too much activity. We all have difficulty saying no to other people, opportunities to serve, demanding work, and even things that would be fun. Some people with chronic pain feel guilty about having to turn down so many opportunities to do enjoyable activities with others. As they begin to recover, they may want to please others, putting their own needs last. Knowing your own limits and keeping to your principles of pacing will help you avoid overcommitting your time and energy.

5. MOVING FORWARD

There is one central message of this book—active pain management is the key to long-term recovery and management of chronic pain. Active pain management means that you are in charge and making the necessary changes in your life to help you move toward health and away from illness and dysfunction.

The alternative to active pain management is a passive approach offered by most healthcare professionals. Passive approaches include the medications, injections, implanted devices, and surgeries prescribed by physicians. People with chronic pain can easily fall prey to the idea that their efforts to recover make no difference when they accept a passive approach to symptom management. When that happens, getting better will seem to be a matter of chance or luck. When successful pain management is only due to chance, we are defeated even before we begin.

One of the most effective coping skills is the mindset of being in charge of one's life. We need to be in the driver's seat, not the passenger seat. Pain needs to be in the passenger seat, or better yet, in the trunk of the car. To develop the attitude and belief that what we do makes a difference, you can practice the following:

- Define what is important to you. What are your values? Who is important to you? What type of character do you want to demonstrate even when facing the challenges of chronic pain?
- Based on your values, set small achievable goals that move you toward what is important to you.
- Expect to have setbacks and failures. When failures occur, be responsible. Responsibility means you learn from your past without blaming yourself, your circumstances, or others. Your choices for how you respond to challenges are your responsibility.
- Evaluate what you are thinking, doing, and feeling, and ask yourself if your behavior is helpful in moving forward and getting your needs met. If your anxiety, fear, anger, bad memories, and frustration are not helpful in bringing about change, then do not feel obligated to hang on to them. Practice letting go, staying present, and moving forward.
- Have positive expectations of good things happening. Remind yourself, "I am okay and am only getting better."

Pay close attention to the pictures you have in your mind of how you picture your life and future. What we picture has a much greater likelihood of coming true.

- Create a new neuromatrix in your brain by following the principles outlined in this book. Managing pain cannot be accomplished by doing one activity or taking one medication. Change how you think, move, view life, handle stress, manage emotions, rest, and react to the sensations your body is sending to your brain. As the individual parts of the neuromatrix change, the brain will dramatically alter how it produces pain.

If you worked through this book on your own, share it with a friend, a family member, or your healthcare professional. Find a supportive individual who will encourage you as you implement the principles and strategies found in this book. Look for an accountability partner who will keep you on task and knows your specific short-term and long-term goals. Join people who are working through chronic pain or other health-related challenges, such as weight loss. Build a team around yourself as you set out to change your relationship with chronic pain. Include your primary care physician in talking through the ideas, research, and concepts presented here. You might be surprised at how supportive healthcare professionals are about hearing that there are good alternatives to managing chronic pain besides the standard approach most physicians use. People like you have faced the same battles you face and have calmed their nervous systems and developed the emotional flexibility to start living again. You can do this, too!

EPILOGUE

I have never in my life envied a human being who led an easy life. I have envied a great many people who led difficult lives and led them well.

—Theodore Roosevelt

Bad things happen to good people all the time. Pain is an unavoidable and inevitable condition of life. If we love others, we will experience pain. If we have hopes and dreams, we will experience pain. As we age, we will experience pain. As we encounter accidents, disease, illness, and injury, we are going to experience pain. Given that we are going to have pain throughout our lives, it seems we have made a huge mistake by not educating people about how the brain produces pain, the value of pain, and how to manage pain so it does not end up controlling our lives.

This book not only provided you with a framework for understanding physical pain but gave you the tools you need to face discomfort, pain, and problems in every area of your life. Think of pain as a classroom instructor who uses a powerful megaphone and yells at us to pay attention. There is a lesson for us to learn in every chapter of our lives. Nothing that happens—good or bad, happy or sad—needs to be wasted in our lives. Those who grow the most and have the most to teach us have gone through the hardest experiences in life and are worthy of our attention and respect.

If you are a chronic pain sufferer, you are one of these people. You have a story to tell and a lesson to teach. The difficult events that have happened in your life have helped you to become a person who is stronger, better, wiser, and kinder. Some of these character changes may have never come about without the difficult challenges that you have experienced and are going through now. You are a remarkable person. Never forget that. You may feel that you do not have much to offer because of your physical or financial condition, but it is not how much you have that matters. What matters is what you do with what you have—your life will leave a mark on those around you. Leave a good one by pouring hope into the lives of those you love.

PATIENT TESTIMONY

As noted in the disclaimer, the three main characters of the book are not real patients. You might wonder if there are real people who make the kind of life changes that are described here. The following is a firsthand account of a former member of the U.S. Special Forces who tried every imaginable treatment for chronic pain without finding relief, just like the characters portrayed in this book. Here is his story in his own words.

REVOLVING DOOR

After a minimum of twenty-four physical therapy programs that included traction, aqua-therapy and Rolfing (some lasting four months), multiple chiropractors, acupuncture, prolotherapy, multiple osteopathic manipulations, special back braces, a plethora of pain creams, gel ice packs, heating pads, a lot of massages, a smorgasbord of non-steroidal anti-inflammatories, high doses of oral steroids, over forty-eight corticosteroid spinal injections, twenty-four spinal nerve blocks, six spinal nerve root rhizotomies, three lumbar surgeries, and a full menu of opioids and benzodiazepines, the low back pain was worse than it had ever been. I saw dozens of doctors, including neurosurgeons, orthopedic surgeons, anesthesiologists, and physiatrists. Full workups were accomplished at the Mayo Clinic in Jacksonville and twice at the Cleveland Clinic. At best, my medical diagnosis—or lack thereof—fell through the cracks of modern medicine. Unable to perform my duties as an AC-130 gunship special operations pilot in the United States Air Force, I was medically retired after twenty-six years.

THE TRANSITION

It seems like I was created just for flying airplanes. I was very good at what I did, and being invincible, there was nothing too difficult for me. I struggled with pain in between missions, but the pain could be managed with healthy doses of ibuprofen and alcohol. It's not as if these social modalities stood out on their own. After flying all night in the supposed cover of darkness, dodging bullets and missiles, it seemed normal to drink myself to sleep. Eventually, my invincibility slowly deteriorated. The downtime from flying missions due to medical intervention became too great. Finally, when the third lumbar surgery made pain conditions unbearable, it was time to face reality. As I was sitting in the chief flight surgeon's office discussing my medical situation, it hit me when he said, "Just how much longer do you think that you want to do this?" It felt like he just slapped me in the head with a brick! Superman does not take kindly to defeat.

THE PERFECT STORM

I was out of a job and unable to work. My income and, more importantly, my identity had been taken away. We moved twice in two years. I had an undiagnosed infection that caused high fevers, uncontrollable shaking, and confusion. Twice, I was hospitalized for septicemia. Out for a walk, I tripped on a trail in the woods and suffered a severe concussion that caused constant headaches and memory problems. To top it off, my perfect job left me suffering from combat-induced post-traumatic stress disorder (PTSD). All the while, I was ingesting 480 mg of morphine and 40 mg of clonazepam daily for pain and anxiety.

I was surprised I was still alive but not necessarily thankful. I was surprised I was still married but not too concerned. If you see your life swirling around the outside edge of a funnel right before it sinks through the center, you are not too concerned with the details!

HERE WE GO AGAIN

I eventually enrolled at Mary Free Bed Rehabilitation Hospital in the pain center. In the back of my head, I knew this was probably my last chance, the end of the road. As I read through the program packet, my eyes fixated on one of the program goals. The plan involved ridding patients of all or most of their pain medication. I focused on the word "most."

The 480 mg of morphine and 40 mg of clonazepam were not working anymore. Prior to this program, I purposely coordinated with my physician to draw down from all medications. I weaned myself down to 30 mg of hydrocodone one month before starting the program and remained at that level through the formal program. For three months, withdrawal symptoms were horrible. Postconcussive symptoms seemed to magnify the withdrawal. I slept for two to three hours a night. Every sixth day, I slept in for a total of four hours. My nervous system felt like it was being shredded. For the first month, I remember cursing Mary Free Bed at home.

YOU GET WHAT YOU GIVE

Military pilots maintain an interesting relationship with their primary care physicians, who are flight surgeons. A flight surgeon can ground a pilot at any time for anything. I learned to talk around some of my issues to keep from getting grounded. A negative behavior pattern I developed was to selectively share information with medical providers. That had proven to be a bad healthcare formula, so I decided instead to be truthful with my healthcare team when I arrived at the Mary Free Bed pain rehabilitation program.

I'll gladly take credit for one thing in this program—I showed up and attended!

I found it extremely important to trust my team and comply with their directions. I implemented every suggestion and homework assignment into daily life as if there was no other choice. My twenty-five-year record of failure in this area dictated program compliance.

What I would normally label "a bunch of crap" helped me lessen withdrawal symptoms and pain. My pain psychologist taught me invaluable lessons in relaxation and mindfulness. I continued to practice the exercises even when I thought they wouldn't help. My medical provider prescribed short-term meds to ease symptoms and, more importantly, listened to me without judgment. It had been a while since someone knowledgeable trusted what I had to say and helped me work through physical issues. My occupational therapist taught me several techniques for enhancing sleep and relaxation. My physical therapist was a master of helping me understand how to best move through life within my circumstances.

MOVING FORWARD WITH LIFE

After graduating from the pain rehabilitation program, I made several follow-up appointments with my pain psychologist, medical provider, nurse, and physical therapist, because that is what I needed to succeed.

Today, I do not use opioids or benzodiazepines (anxiety medication)!

I encountered several new setbacks while enrolled in the program. The muddy waters, created by all the medication, began to clear up and reveal other physical and emotional problems. Both my hips and one knee were surgically repaired. Six teeth were extracted for infection, and an extensive oral surgery session paved the way for future dental implants. The oral bone grafts required that I quit smoking. After forty years of using nicotine, I used mindfulness exercises to quit without looking back.

Some very negative behavior patterns from my PTSD developed due to long-term exposure to significant physical and emotional

events. These negative behavior patterns resulted in significant rela-
tionship problems. Without relationships, the soul crumbles. My pain
psychologist guided me through the release of emotional pain and
paranoia associated with traumatic memories.

My very patient wife and I have been married thirty-six years.
Prior to this program, I knew our relationship was severely strained,
but I was mentally unequipped to effect any positive change.

Today, our marriage is like the adventuresome experience we had
dating in high school, enjoying the moment, not sweating the small
stuff.

I now sleep for five to seven hours a night!

Instead of pain medication, I use the toolbox given to me by my
healthcare team at Mary Free Bed every day.

Today, I'm not mad at anyone or anything. I'm certainly more
compassionate for those experiencing some type of duress. Most
importantly, at the beginning of each day, I become excited at the
prospect of making someone laugh!

WHAT IS YOUR STORY?

After reading this short account of one person's journey from
being stuck in chronic pain to moving forward with life, maybe
you would like to share your own story of how you are able to
manage pain. You can share your story by going to my website,
PainRehabSource.com, and clicking on the link to submit your
story. Your story will then be featured on the website and then
serve as an encouragement to others. I am looking forward to
hearing from you!

RESOURCE ONE: THE BIG PICTURE

Pain is a distressing experience associated with actual or perceived tissue damage with sensory, emotional, cognitive, and social components.

—The International Association for the Study of Pain

There are several important elements of the International Association for the Study of Pain's (IASP) definition of pain. Pain may be related to actual tissue damage, like a cut, or it can occur when there is no injury at all. There are also many factors that influence the perception of pain, including what we think, our past experiences, the context of our current circumstances, our emotions, and the overall condition of our nervous system. The

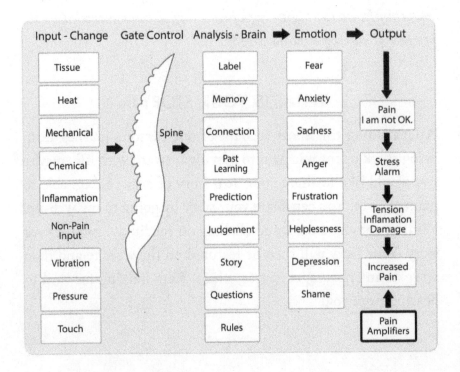

brain receives information from the sensory, motor, emotional, cognitive, and behavioral parts of the nervous system and is organized by the brain's neuromatrix. The brain produces pain when it determines there is evidence of a threat based on the organization and information contained in the neuromatrix.

The IASP definition of pain is very good, but it is also a challenge for us to understand how all those different elements work together. The model presented in this book focuses on the role of the central nervous system (brain and spinal cord). The central nervous system can become overly sensitive so that almost any activity (any type of sensory input) will be reacted to as if it is a threat. The brain is constantly looking for credible evidence of danger and credible evidence of safety. When the analysis weighs in favor of danger and threat, then the brain will produce pain in order to warn and protect us. An overly sensitive nervous system is like a motion detector that is set incorrectly and goes off at the slightest movement in a yard or room. Likewise, everything that changes in the body—even the touch on the skin—ends up feeding into the evidence of danger, and the brain keeps producing pain.

It is often difficult for us to accept that pain is not solely something that happens because of injury or damage. We wrongly picture pain coming from our nerve endings traveling up to the brain, rather than realizing that the nerve endings only send information about changes that have occurred, not pain. This explanation of how the brain produces pain is critical when thinking about how chronic pain develops. For example, a person with chronic regional pain syndrome (CRPS) can go to bed one night with the CRPS symptoms in the right leg and wake up in the morning with the symptoms transferred to the left leg. This does not occur because the nerves in the left leg were mysteriously damaged in the night. Only by looking at how the entire nervous system operates and becomes overly sensitive can we see how the psychological, social, and biological dimensions are interconnected and each have roles in the production of chronic pain.

The model provided in this book has four main elements: (1) input from the sensory nerves; (2) analysis by the brain; (3) the brain's output, which is the sensation of pain; and (4) the role of stress and other factors that can amplify pain. The four common signs that a person has shifted from acute to chronic pain include: (1) pain spreading and changing locations; (2) heightened sensitivity to non-pain sensory input, such as a light touch, breezes, temperature changes, or vibrations; (3) changes in the experience of pain from dull and aching to burning, stabbing, throbbing, numb, or tingling; and (4) pain that is out of proportion with the injury experienced.

As the central nervous system becomes overly sensitive, the role of input from the sensory nerves becomes less important. Once the brain is constantly evaluating everything as a threat and is collecting more evidence of danger than of safety, even in the absence of a significant physical change or threat, the brain will still produce chronic pain. Effective chronic pain management involves calming down the central nervous system and changing how the brain is wired so that new pathways are formed that do not link pain with movement.

RESOURCE TWO:
THE PROBLEM WITH OPIOID MEDICATIONS

The Center For Disease Control (CDC) issues guidelines that help physicians know what types of treatment and medication are helpful for treating certain medical conditions and which are not helpful. Specific guidelines have been given regarding the use of opioid medications to treat chronic pain. The first guideline states, "Nonpharmacologic therapy and nonopioid therapy are preferred for chronic pain."[1.] The CDC's key recommendation suggests that treatments not involving medications are the best approach to use when treating chronic pain.

The CDC guidelines are important because of the new research that shows others that opioid medications are not helpful for chronic pain, even though they can be useful for short-term (acute) pain. Opioids, possibly due to aggressive advertising, are viewed by many healthcare professionals and patients alike as an effective treatment for chronic pain. This has led to a serious problem in overprescribing opioids for managing pain, which has caused both federal and state governments to make it harder to prescribe the medications.

A common path toward the ongoing use of opioid medication is to have it first prescribed for acute pain management after surgery or serious injury. With acute pain, opioids can be effective in managing pain. Unfortunately, after the normal period of healing has passed, opioid medications are sometimes continued. This presents a serious problem. Opioid medications, like alcohol, lead to both tolerance and dependence. Once a person takes an opioid medication for months or years, the use of the medication cannot easily be stopped without experiencing difficult and very uncomfortable withdrawal symptoms. This is the result of a person becoming dependent on the opioid—their body needs the medication to function. If a person attempts to go off their opioid medication on their own, they can have dangerous medical complications.

The tolerance of opioids is also a significant problem. Because of tolerance to opioid medications, the dosage must be increased over time to keep providing some type of benefit. A person might take a low dosage once a day for acute pain but will eventually take higher doses several times a day one year later; they are attempting to get the same benefit of pain relief that the low dosage once provided. With increased amounts of opioids in the body, problems soon develop with how the brain and internal organs function, and chronic pain is made significantly worse.

HOW OPIOIDS WORK IN THE BRAIN

The brain is in charge of keeping us safe. In order to keep us safe, the brain needs information about the body, inside and out. We have forty-three miles of peripheral nerves feeding into the central nervous system (brain and spinal cord). As information comes to the brain regarding change and damage (e.g., you sprained your ankle), the brain can produce natural opioids and reduce our pain. But when a person takes an opioid medication for a long period of time, the brain's natural ability to produce opioids is shut down. Opioids should be produced by our brain and used to manage and run many other functions in the body besides pain management. Turning off the brain's natural opioid production produces unwanted side effects and makes life difficult for the person taking the medication.

When a person is taking an opioid medication, the brain's ability to get information about what is happening in the body is reduced.[2.] To picture this problem of reduced information, imagine putting on an ear protection headset like the ear protection airport workers use near airplanes. Opioids limit information getting to the brain and muffle sensory input like the ear protection headset; opioids block out information that the brain is trying to get about what is happening in the body. The brain wants to know: Is that knee working well? How is the back today? What is going on with the neck? Due to the information-blocking ability of the opioid medication, the brain is robbed of the information it needs.

The brain creates a wonderful solution to this problem by producing *more pain receptors* since the ones that it normally has are being blocked by the opioid medication. As the brain produces more pain receptors, the brain then becomes much more sensitive to every type of sensation, movement, change, and activity that occurs throughout the body. As the brain produces more pain receptors, pain can spread and intensify, making chronic pain worse.

OPIOIDS CAN MAKE PAIN WORSE

Without realizing the risk involved, opioids that have been prescribed for acute pain end up playing a role in the development of chronic pain due to the medication's impact on the brain. As awareness of this problem is increasing, changes are being made in how chronic pain is being approached by physicians. New non-opioid medications are being used, but the most important change has come in the recognition that many people can learn to manage pain and reduce their pain even with little or no use of any type of medication.

To help with these changes, healthcare professionals need to talk with their patients about their reliance on opioids for pain management. There needs to be a long conversation with the patient about why this approach is important. The conversation might go like this:

The physician asks, "I see you have been on a high dose of morphine for several years. Do you think this is helping you?"

The patient replies, "Oh yes. I cannot function without it, but I am still in a great deal of pain."

"If you are in a great deal of pain, maybe the morphine is not doing what you think it is."

"What do you mean? I can barely move if I miss a dose of my medication."

"Yes. You have not been moving very much in several years because of your pain. With or without medication, movement is going to be difficult for you. It really does not look like you are benefiting from the medication. Plus, you have many other side effects from morphine that are impacting your ability to think, have energy to function, and control your emotions."

"Oh yes. I often take Extra Strength Tylenol for my headaches I get about once a week. The Tylenol helps a lot."

"So you are on enough daily morphine that would knock out the average person for three days, but you have to take Tylenol for a headache? If your morphine is effective, why do you think you need to take Tylenol?"

"Now that you put it like that, I am not sure. Maybe the morphine isn't really helping."

"You are correct. The morphine is not helping you manage your pain at all."

Once a patient like this is weaned off the morphine, which is a challenging, slow process in itself, positive changes begin to occur. First, the patient is able to think clearly. While on opioids, the mind often feels like it is in a fog, and it is hard to focus and recall information. This changes quickly as opioids are reduced. Secondly, the normal functioning of the intestines begins to return. Third, the sleep-wake cycle improves. Patients are less tired during the day, stop napping, and sleep better at night, which improves many other important emotional and physical processes. In addition, sexual functioning and other hormone-regulated functions are restored as normal hormonal functioning is regulated naturally by the body. It will take time, months in some cases, to get all the opioids out of a person's system, but gradually a person will begin to feel clear-headed and able to function once again.

I AM NOT A DRUG ADDICT

Patients are understandably upset about the changes occurring in medicine due to the opioid crisis. For years or even decades, patients with chronic pain were prescribed opioid medications. They faithfully took their pain medications just like any other medication that would be prescribed for blood pressure or cholesterol. These same patients are now going to their doctors and being told that they should not be taking opioids. Some patients are even treated by their healthcare providers as if they are "drug-seeking" problem patients. At times, patients need to find new primary care physicians because their doctors refused to have such "risky" patients on opioids on their caseloads. This leaves the patient desperate for help and answers. It is heartbreaking to hear a 75-year-old patient say, "I am not a drug addict! I have been prescribed this medication for twenty years, and now I am being treated like a criminal."

There is clearly not enough information being provided to healthcare professionals and patients alike about good alternatives to opioid medications. The information provided in this book is designed specifically to help outline an approach to understanding and managing chronic pain that is being successfully used in multidisciplinary rehabilitation treatment programs around the country and internationally.

ENDNOTES

CHAPTER ONE

1. Dubin, A., & Patapoultian, A. (2010). 'Nociceptors: The sensors of the pain pathway'. *Journal of Clinical Investigation, 120*(11), 3760–3772.
2. Schaible, H. G., & Richter F. (2004). 'Pathophysiology of pain'. *Langenbeck's Archives of Surgery, 389*(4), 237–243.

CHAPTER TWO

1. Mosely, G. L., & Butler, D. S. (2015). *The explain pain handbook: Protectometer.* South Africa: Noigroup Publications.
2. Creamer P., & Hockburg, M. C. (1997). 'Why does osteoarthritis of the knee hurt—Sometimes?' *Britsh Journal of Rheumatology, 36*(7), 726–728.
3. Louw, A., Diener, I., Fernández-de-Las-Peñas. C., & Puente-dura E. J. (2016). 'Sham surgery in orthopedics: A systematic review of the literature'. *Pain Medicine, 18(*4), 736–750.

CHAPTER SEVEN

1. Coughlin, S. S. (2012). 'Anxiety and depression: Linkages with viral diseases'. *Public Health Review, 34*(2), 92.

2. Klein, T. W. (1993). 'Stress and Infections'. *Journal of the Florida Medical Association, 80*(6), 409–411.

3. U.S. Department of Health and Human Services Office on Women's Health. (2019). *Autoimmune Diseases Fact Sheet.*

CHAPTER NINE

1. Moayedi, M., Davis, K. D. (2012). 'Theories of pain: From specificity to gate control'. *Journal of Neurophysiology, 109*(1), 5–12.

CHAPTER TEN

1. Kerns, R. D., Otis, J. D., & Wise, E. A. (2002). 'Treating families of chronic pain patients'. In D.C. Tuck & R.J. Catchel (Eds.) *Psychological approaches to pain management. (2nd ed.)* (pp. 105-123). New York, NY: Guilford Press.

2. Wilson, S. J., Martire, L. M., & Sliwinski, M. J. (2017). 'Daily spousal responsiveness predicts longer-term trajectories of patients' physical function'. *Psychological Science, 28*(6), 786.

CHAPTER ELEVEN

1. Mosely, G. L., & Butler, D. S. (2015). *The explain pain handbook: Protectometer.* South Africa: Noigroup Publications.

2. Herzog, R. (2017). 'Variability in diagnostic error rates in 10 MRI centers performing lumbar spine MRI examinations on the same patient within the three-week period'. *Spine Journal,17*, 554–561.

3. Chou, R., Qaseem, A., Snow, V., Casey, D., Cross, J. T., Shekelle, P., & Owens, D. J. (2007). 'Diagnosis and treatment of low back pain: A joint clinical practice guideline from the American College of Physicians and the American Pain Society'. *Annals of Internal Medicine, 147*(7), 478-491.

4. Brinjiki, W., Luetmer, P. H., Comstock, B., Bresnahan, B. W., Chen, L. E., Deyo, R. A., Halabi, S., Turner, J. A., Avins, A. L., Wald, J. T., Kallmes, D. F., & Jarvik, J. G. (2015). 'Systematic literature review of imaging features of spinal degeneration in asymptomatic populations'. *American Journal of Neuroradiology, 36,* 811–816

5. Deyo, R. A. (2007). 'Back surgery: Who needs it?' *New England Journal of Medicine, 356,* 2239–2243

6. Nguyen, T. H., Randolph, D. C., Talmage, J., Succop, P., & Travis, R. (2011). 'Long-term outcomes of lumbar fusion among workers' compensation subjects: a historical cohort study'. *Spine, 36*(4), 320–31.

7. Louw, A., Diener, I., Fernández-de-Las-Peñas, C., Puentedura, E. J. (2016). 'Sham surgery in orthopedics: A systematic review of the literature'. *Pain Medicine, 18(*4), 736–750.

CHAPTER TWELVE

1. Butler, D. S., & Moseley, G. L. (2013). *Explain pain* (2nd ed.). Adelaide, South Australia: Noigroup Publication.

CHAPTER THIRTEEN

1. Ecsy, K., Jones, A. K. P., & Brown, C. A. (2017). 'Alpha-range visual and auditory stimulation reduces the perception of pain'. *European Journal of Pain, 21,* 562–572.

CHAPTER FIFTEEN

1. Anspaugh, D. J., Hamrick, M. H., & Rosato, F. D. (2011). *Wellness: Concepts and applications* (8th ed.). New York, NY: McGraw-Hill Education.

CHAPTER SIXTEEN

1. Rozenberg, S., Allaert, F. A., Savarieau, B., Perahia, M., & Valat, J. P. (2004). 'Compliance among general practitioners in France with recommendations not to prescribe bed rest for acute low back pain'. *Joint Bone Spine, 71*(1), 56–59.
2. Cooney, J. K., Law, R., Matschke, V., Lemmey, A. B., Moore, J. P., Ahmad, Y., Jones, J. G., Maddison, P., & Thom, J. M. (2011). 'Benefits of exercise in rheumatoid arthritis'. *Journal of Aging Research, 2011*, 681–640.

CHAPTER SEVENTEEN

1. Polk, K. L., & Schoendorff, B. (Eds.). (2014). *The ACT Matrix: A new approach to building psychological flexibility across settings and populations*. Oakland, CA: New Harbinger Publications.

CHAPTER EIGHTEEN

1. McCracken, L. M., & Vowles, K. E. (2014). 'Acceptance and commitment therapy and mindfulness for chronic pain: Model, process, and progress'. *American Psychologist, 69*(2), 178–187.

CHAPTER NINETEEN

1. Harris, R. (2019). *ACT made simple*. Oakland, CA: New Harbinger Publications.
2. Thompson, M., & McCracken, L. (2011). 'Acceptance and related processes in adjustment to chronic pain'. *Current Pain and Headache Reports, 15*, 144–151.

CHAPTER TWENTY

1. Harris, R. (2019). *ACT made simple.* Oakland, CA: New Harbinger Publications.
2. Polk, K. L., & Schoendorff, B. (Eds.) (2014) *The ACT matrix: A new approach to building psychological flexibility across settings and populations.* Oakland, CA: New Harbinger Publications.
3. Hayes, S. (2005). *Get out of your mind and into your life: The new acceptance and commitment therapy.* Oakland. CA: New Harbinger Publications.

CHAPTER TWENTY-ONE

1. Hayes, S. (2005). *Get out of your mind and into your life: The new acceptance and commitment therapy.* Oakland. CA: New Harbinger Publications.
2. Harris, R. (2008). *The happiness trap: How to stop struggling and start living: A guide to ACT.* Durban, South Africa: Trumpeter.
3. Harris, R. (2019). *ACT made simple.* Oakland, CA: New Harbinger Publications.

REFERENCES

1. CDC Guideline for Prescribing Opioids for Chronic Pain—United States, 2016.
2. Lee, M., Silverman, S. M., Hansen, H., Patel, V. B., & Manchikanti, L. (2011). 'A comprehensive review of opioid-induced hyperalgesia'. *Pain Physician, 14*(2): 145-161.

ACKNOWLEDGEMENTS

The story of this book's inception begins with the chronic pain patients I see every day. The courage, dedication, and hope that they display, often in the face of challenging life circumstances, is a constant source of inspiration for me. Their stories of struggle—along with the amazing, transformative changes that take place when they approach their pain differently—have shaped my knowledge of the brain's neuromatrix map.

However, for all the chronic patients that I have been able to meet and help, there are thousands more who will never receive the kind of medical care that they need and deserve. Perhaps the isolation of a rural community prevents access to care, or maybe all the hours of the day are spent working two jobs and raising children, leaving no time to care for themselves.

Regardless of the reason, I want the knowledge of how the nervous system operates and how chronic pain is managed to be understood—both by those suffering *and* by those caring for them. *What should be common knowledge is not.* Despite living in an age of information and advertising overload, there is a disconnect: no real improvement in the human condition.

It is my greatest hope that this book will help the reader cut through the noise, hear something that makes sense, and get back to living a life they love. You—dear reader—are my reason for writing. Thank you.

Lastly, to my wife, Carrie. We had no idea the adventures we would go on together! From the very beginning of our life together, to raising our children in Budapest, Hungary, to helping those in harm's way in many different countries, you have always been my partner and companion. Without your support and encouragement, I would not be the person I am today. When all I see are problems, you always see what is good, useful, and true.

INDEX

Page numbers in **bold** refer to illustrations.

biopsychosocial approach ix, 90–2
bitterness 96–7
blame 232
blood circulation 61, 145, 253
blood flow 167
blood pressure 83, 148
body awareness 153–64
  awareness and attention 156–7
  mindfulness body scan 155–64
  noticing 157–8
bone-on-bone damage 22–3
brain 7, 252–3
  and acceptance 227
  attention-getting devices 224
  busy 150
  calming 150
  conditioning 19, 258
  danger-in-me (DIM) scale
    118–19, 120–2, 253, 255
  fear of movement 180
  functions 58–9
  information accuracy 82, 118–19
  job 222
  lack of information 41
  meaning making 30
  monitoring systems 32–3
  neuroplasticity 8
  news media outlet metaphor
    222–3
  noise 186–7
  opioid impacts 270–1
  output reduction 249
  oversensitized 103
  oxygen supply 144
  pain production 34, 35–6, **36**
  pain response 14, 267
  pain scale balance 116–18, **117**
  pain sensation 29–30

rehearsal 126–7
reprogramming 36
role of 35
safety-in-me (SIM) scale
  119–20, 125–7, 253, 255
storytelling powers 222–3
stress response 61
thanking 223
threat evaluation 21–2, 23,
  30–2, 34, 55–6, 105–14, 249,
  267–8
threat perception 81, 84
warning alarms 32–3, 34
word-machine metaphor 222
brain analysis, and emotions
  55–6, **55**
brain chemistry 93
brain input analysis 34, 35–6, **43**
  cause connection 38–9
  judgment 40–1
  lack of information 41
  and memory 37–8
  past learning 39–40
  prediction 40, 44, 127–8
  questions 42–3
  rules 43–5, 126
  sense making 39
  sensory experience labelling 36–7
  and story 42
brain wave activity, changing
  149–50
breathing cycle 147
breathing exercises 125, 127, 129,
  240
  diaphragmatic breathing
    145–52, 254
  progressive muscle relaxation
    (PMR) 171, 173

breathing power 148–9
breathing rate 144–5
Butler, David 117–18

caffeine 82, 154, 229, 232, 234
Caleb case study 17–19
calming strategies 254
Center For Disease Control
(CDC) 269
central nervous system 14, 20–1,
59, **60**, 267–8
electrical activity 108
floodlight metaphor 107
motion detector metaphor 107
sensitization signs 84–8
central sensitization 8, 84–8,
267–8
change 212–13
barriers to 203
waiting for trap 247
chemical coping 229
chemical detection nerves 28
chemical messengers 33
choice, sense of 201
choices
moving forward 247–8
paying attention to 241
Christine case study 38–9, 40
chronic pain
conceptualization 15–16
development of 17–19
Chronic Pain and Fatigue
Research Center 22
chronic regional pain syndrome
(CRPS) 267–8
chronic stress 57
diagnosis 70–3
doctor recommendations 73–4

immune response during 62–4
impact 71
impact on mind 70
Rachel case study 67–74
symptoms 67–70, 72
classical conditioning 16–19, **17,
18**, 40
Clauw, Daniel 22–3
commitment 186–7
commonsense assumptions 26
conditioning 16–19, **17, 18**, 40
control 201–2, 220, 220–1, 234,
239
lack of 48, 49, 191–4
loss of 98–9
and suffering 194
cooldown exercises 185–6
corticotropin releasing hormone
(CRH) 61–2
cortisol 63, 83
cramping 170
credibility 12
credible evidence 21–2
cytokines 63

daily activities
pacing 139–42
planning 174
danger-in-me (DIM) 118–19,
120–2, 180, 253, 255
David case study 3, 89–90, 90–1,
251
acceptance 224–7
anger 96
anxiety 98–9
bitterness 96–7
condition of nervous system 7
expectation setting 132–3

withdrawal symptoms 270
opting out 232–3
outside world 196

pacing 134–5, **135**, 137–9, **138, 139**, 255–6
  exercise 184–5
  practice of 140–2
pain
  accepting 20
  anticipated 16
  approach to 6–9
  classroom instructor metaphor 259–60
  experience of ix, 15–16
  fear of 78–9
  IASP definition 266–7
  inevitability of 259
  label change 85, 87
  location change 87–8
  location of 27–30, **29**
  as motivator 251–2
  perception of 16, 266
  purpose of 32, 32–3
  reality of 25
  and small events 26
  stopping talking about 110
  understanding 252–3, 266–8, **266**
  see also acute pain
pain acceptance 157, 163, 181
pain alarm 14
pain amplifiers 89–101, **91**
  anger 96
  anxiety 98–9
  bitterness 96–7
  David case study 89–90, 90–1
  electric guitar metaphor 91–2

  fear 97–8
  loneliness 99–100
  reframing 100–1
  sadness 99
  stress 95
pain behavior 213
pain catastrophizing 79–80
pain creams 79
pain education 19–20, 22
pain intensity 110–11
  and degree of injury 22–3, 25–7
pain levels 52, 111
pain management 6, 81, 90, 113–14, 252, 253
  active 114, 256–8
  automatic 201
  effective 114
  focusing on 50
  passive 113–14, 256–7
  and suffering 191–3
pain nerves 29
pain patches 79
pain pathways, reactivation of old 76–7
pain perception 92–3, **94**
pain production, in the brain 34, 35–6, **36**
pain receptors 271
pain reducers 202
pain response, brain 14
pain scale balance 116–18, **117**, 127–9, **129**
  danger-in-me (DIM) 118–19, 120–2
  safety-in-me (SIM) 119–20, 125–7
pain sensitivity 82, 154

ABOUT THE AUTHOR

Dr. Evan Parks is a clinical psychologist working in pain reha-bilitation at Mary Free Bed Rehabilitation Hospital and is an adjunct assistant professor at Michigan State University College of Human Medicine. He is committed to helping people move toward well-being and away from physical and emotional problems that get in the way of a rich and rewarding life. He spent fifteen years working in Eastern Europe teaching principles of mental health and responding to crisis situations throughout the region. Along the way, he learned to appreciate how different cultures and demographics deal with pain and mental health problems.